"This book is the culmination of many years of clinical experience of providing psychotherapy to women experiencing perinatal mental distress. Emma's wisdom and compassion flow from the page and as you will see, her writing style is clear, accessible, and 'speaks to' not only the reader, but to the very women she is writing about. Haynes has provided our profession with a handbook for the psychotherapy of maternal mental illness that all psychotherapists- regardless of their theoretical orientation or modality can make use of. I am certain that many readers – myself included – will keep this book to hand and return to it often as a trusted practical guide when working with women who are experiencing perinatal mental health problems."
Mark Widdowson, *UKCP Registered Psychotherapist, Senior lecturer in counselling and psychotherapy, University of Salford, UK*

Motherhood and Mental Illness

Motherhood and Mental Illness offers an in-depth, comprehensive relational psychotherapeutic framework to provide effective treatment for those experiencing maternal mental illness.

This book addresses a current deficit in mental health resources and treatment and is designed to be an accessible, practical guide to the types and manifests of disorders and the diagnosis, treatment and management of maternal mental illness. It gives a solid understanding of the nature and complexity of maternal mental illness and offers clear guidance on how to provide treatment for successful recovery. Then, using a relational approach, the book offers useful therapeutic interventions grounded in clinical experience and research, which are elucidated with case examples. Covering the most common presentations and the confounders (alcohol, single parenting, drug abuse, self-medication) this is a guide of how to plan treatment, common mistakes that can occur, myths that prevail, and ethical dilemmas.

The book will be suitable for psychotherapists and counsellors of any modality as well as any healthcare professionals who have frontline contact with women.

Emma Haynes, PhD, is a Teaching and Supervising Transactional Analyst and UKCP-registered psychotherapist who has dedicated her professional life to researching and treating maternal mental illness and developmental trauma. She is a lecturer in psychotherapy at Metanoia Institute, London.

Motherhood and Mental Illness

A Relational Treatment Approach

Emma Haynes

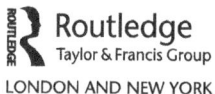

Routledge
Taylor & Francis Group

LONDON AND NEW YORK

Cover image: © Getty Images.

First published 2023
by Routledge
4 Park Square, Milton Park, Abingdon, Oxon OX14 4RN

and by Routledge
605 Third Avenue, New York, NY 10158

Routledge is an imprint of the Taylor & Francis Group, an informa business

British Library Cataloguing-in-Publication Data
A catalogue record for this book is available from the British Library

Library of Congress Cataloging-in-Publication Data
A catalog record has been requested for this book

ISBN: 9780367724627 (hbk)
ISBN: 9780367724610 (pbk)
ISBN: 9781003154891 (ebk)

DOI: 10.4324/9781003154891

Typeset in Bembo
by KnowledgeWorks Global Ltd.

To my clients, and all the other mothers
in the world: speak out, we can hear you.

This book is dedicated to the memory
of Miriam Edmond, a superb midwife who
was utterly dedicated to the women she
cared for. A huge loss to midwifery.

Contents

Figures

Foreword

One afternoon, in September 2014, I received an email from a psychotherapist who wanted to talk to me about my research on the effectiveness of transactional analysis (TA) for depression. The psychotherapist was Emma Haynes, the author of this book, and she wanted to talk to me about how TA might help women with postnatal depression. The email exchange quickly evolved and within a matter of weeks Emma had started her PhD at the University of Salford and I was her research supervisor. Each month, she made the long drive from her home close to the south coast of England up to Greater Manchester for doctoral supervision meetings. In the weeks between our meetings, she would trawl through databases of research, looking for articles which addressed maternal mental health, and would produce several thousand word summaries of these articles and bring them with her to our next meeting. I can still recall feeling shocked and deeply unsettled to discover just how common mental health problems are for women in the perinatal period and also just how little there is in the way of treatment for them to access. These were *pregnant women* and *women with small babies*, for heaven's sake. Surely there must be *something* for them? Therapy services seemed very thin on the ground, hard to access, and therapy that was on offer was often too short to be of real solid help. Medication was not usually an option, and even when it was, women were usually understandably afraid of taking it for fear of harming their babies. Realising that what was on offer was only scratching the surface and that each day many thousands of women are struggling alone was a disturbing thought. Despite the fact that protecting pregnant women and women with newborns is very likely to be woven into the deepest recesses of our psyche as an ancient survival mechanism for our entire species, we let them down, and we let them down badly. This is a hard truth to face.

Emma identified themes in the many obstacles these women faced. Mostly, they would not only be struggling with their mental health, but they would be deeply afraid. Frightened not only by what they were experiencing, but terrified about what might happen if they told anyone how they were feeling. Would their children be taken away from them? Would they be branded unfit mothers? What on Earth would people think of them? Here the often unspoken pressures on women to be perfect and the thinly veiled misogyny that runs deep through our societies seemed to be a major driving force, fuelling their terror.

Over the coming years, a different, more optimistic tone started to emerge as Emma's data, taken from interviews with women who had received psychotherapy for perinatal mental health problems, started to show that healing was possible. As Emma went deeper into the data and the narratives of the women she had interviewed, she identified a more nuanced picture highlighting that the key to change (like with many psychotherapies) was in the therapeutic relationship, and that it seemed that the most potent change occurred through the use of relational psychotherapy.

This book is the culmination of Emma's PhD, her ongoing study and research into maternal mental health, and her many years of clinical experience providing psychotherapy to women experiencing perinatal mental distress. Her wisdom and compassion flow from the page and as you will see, her writing style is clear, accessible, and 'speaks to' not only the reader, but to the very women she is writing about.

In Chapter 1, *Transitions*, Emma paints a vivid picture of the transition to motherhood, and how some women find that the transition is not the happy event that they had hoped and planned for. In Chapter 2, *A Silent Problem*, we start to get a sense as to the magnitude and complexity of the problem that is maternal mental illness. Haynes accounts for the psychological factors, as well as biological aspects associated with pregnancy and motherhood and the sociocultural forces that form an intricate web around and throughout all of our lives, and the impact these have on new mothers, mothers to be, and women who are already mothers who are having another child. Chapter 3, *Historical Aspects of Maternal Mental Illness*, takes us on a deeply disturbing journey of the pathologising of women experiencing perinatal mental health problems and the sexism and inequality that is embedded within society that influences – even to this day – how these women are treated by health professionals and viewed within society. Haynes broadens our view in Chapter 4: Pre-Conception, Common Conditions and Confounders, where she explores some of the different ways in which perinatal mental distress is experienced and many of the issues women with these experiences are likely to present with in our therapy rooms. The impact of the currently ongoing COVID-19 pandemic is considered here, and how lockdowns and 'working from home' rules have changed childcare and gender roles. The issue of *Maternal Trauma* is discussed in Chapter 5, where Haynes discusses a number of traumatic circumstances which can generate or feed into perinatal mental health problems. Each type of trauma is considered from the point of view of both the woman and the therapist, with implications for how these might be addressed in therapy made clear. We are once again taken deeper in Chapter 6, which explores *Postpartum Psychosis* – the most severe type of maternal mental illness. Haynes does not shy away from explaining to us the true horrors of postpartum psychosis. However, the chapter – like the others in this book – retains a sense of hopefulness, a sense that new meaning can be found and that healing and growth is possible. Chapter 7 presents *Narratives of Maternal Mental Illness,* where Haynes introduces the reader to the themes she has identified in her research and in her practice, which infuse the narratives of the women who are seeking therapy. It is hard to overstate just how useful this will be to the practicing therapists who each day sit in their consulting rooms, trying to help women make sense of their experiences as they co-construct meaning. The many *Barriers to Treatment* are explored in Chapter 8. This is another thought-provoking read, and one which therapists and services would do well to consider in figuring out how collectively we can make this journey easier for women, and in helping us to understand some of what they have had to overcome (and continue to battle with) to actually manage to arrive in our offices and sit in front of us, seeking our help. We are introduced to *A Relational Approach* in Chapter 9. As Haynes is writing through a relational lens in the whole book, we get a sense of something which is comfortable and familiar and of a framework which ties together the many disparate and often tangled threads we have, laid before us. The very real and many *Ethical Dilemmas in Motherhood* and in providing therapy to perinatal women are explored in their gritty realism in Chapter 10. The reader is offered a series of questions for further reflection and exploration as Haynes wisely and resolutely refuses to provide rigid and pre-determined one-size-fits-all solutions to what are always complex, nuanced and individualised situations. In Chapter 11, we consider Treating the *Treating the Cause of Maternal Mental Illness* by looking at some of the historical antecedents and underlying factors which affect mental health, and which create vulnerabilities which can be exposed in their rawness when a woman becomes pregnant and/or has a baby. The issue of *Affect Regulation* is considered in Chapter 12. Over the years, I have come to the view that almost all mental illnesses and mental health problems are issues of affect regulation. The importance of affect regulation for the mother is highlighted here and is presented once again in a way that offers the practicing therapist much food for thought and grist for the therapeutic mill. In Chapter 13, the reader is taken back to the therapeutic relationship to consider what is their *Therapeutic Role* for their client. The chapter is infused with modern attachment theory and insights from the world of relational psychoanalysis. Working *Using Creativity and Creative Methods in Psychotherapy* is explored in Chapter 14 as a means to both enrich the therapeutic process, and also as a method to unlock and explore the many layers of unconscious process our clients bring into the room. Many readers, like myself, will be pleased to see the issue of *Neurodivergence and Motherhood* considered in Chapter 15. An increasing number of therapists are realising that our traditional ways of working do not adequately serve the therapeutic needs of clients who are neurodivergent. The implications for therapy are explored and practical tips are offered to the reader to help them adjust how they work with neurodivergent clients. *Couples Work* is refreshingly discussed in Chapter 16. Given that most babies are born to parents who are in relationships, and that mental illness in one partner will inevitably affect the other, exploration of couples therapy is a strong addition to this book. Chapter 17: Conventional Treatment of Maternal Mental Illness provides the reader with a helpful overview of conventional medical treatment for depression and postpartum mental illness. For non-medically trained psycho-therapists, such summaries are useful for a basic understanding of medication and, in the case of perinatal mental health problems, the potential issues of harm to the fetus or newborn. Finally, in Chapter 18: A Lifetime Reduction in Mental Illness?, Haynes takes up a clarion call for us to consider the wider social and transgenerational impact of providing adequate care and appro-priate psychotherapy for maternal mental illness and its potential role in pre-venting mental health problems for future generations.

Haynes has provided our profession with a handbook for the psychother-apy of maternal mental illness that all psychotherapists – regardless of their theoretical orientation or modality can make use of. I am certain that many readers – myself included – will keep this book to hand and return to it often as a trusted practical guide when working with women who are experiencing perinatal mental health problems.

Dr Mark Widdowson
UKCP Registered Psychotherapist
Senior Lecturer in Counselling and Psychotherapy
University of Salford, Manchester
January 2022

Preface: Seeds of Life

Sat at my desk, writing this introduction, I am reflecting on the thrill of beginning a new journey and the developmental process from planting a single tiny seed, watching it spring into life and seeing it develop through the wonder of evolution. Journeys, transitions and development are underlying themes in this book. When I first began my journey into perinatal mental illness, I was a trainee psychotherapist, needing clinical experience at the sharp end of mental health for my postgraduate degree and UK Council of Psychotherapy (UKCP) accreditation. I didn't realise that my first moment in a mother and baby in-patient psychiatric unit (MBU) would plant the seed that would develop into my entire professional career. Stern, Bruschweiler-Stern and Freeland draw attention to the change in women from the moment of conception 'In the course of becoming a mother, […], a woman develops a mindset fundamentally different from the one she held before, and enters a realm of experience not known to non-mothers' (1998, p. 5). In much the same way, I also was fundamentally changing.

From the moment I walked into the MBU I became passionate and also angry. Passionate to help the women and their families with the awfulness that is maternal mental illness, and in particular postpartum psychosis. Angry because, at the time, there was no psychological help offered to these women, either in the unit, or after discharge. When I was asked to stop giving therapy, in case it began a precedence that someone (the health service) would then need to pay for, this anger became determination. The determination then became organisation. Firstly, I knew that I would not be taken seriously unless I increased my knowledge and experience, so I chose to do a PhD researching transactional analysis (TA) as a treatment for perinatal mental illness. I also knew that no matter how long I worked, I could not treat everyone. In fact, I was more useful teaching other therapists to work in this area. If I limited myself only to client work, then the knowledge I had gained would not disseminate in the way it needs to. I needed to begin to fill the black hole of research into this illness and into psychotherapy as an effective and suitable alternative to psychotropic medication. Maternal mental illness is like a black hole of nothingness, and the lack of psychotherapeutic help is like a gaping chasm:

- It is a black hole of distress, silence and shame.
- There is little in the way of help specific to motherhood.
- There is a gaping hole in research, although it is finally beginning to be addressed, albeit glacially slowly, through a growing number of research projects into areas such as miscarriage and infant loss, working with neurodiversity, difference and diversity.
- There is a lack of basic knowledge and understanding in the medical profession and wider society about this illness.
- There is a serious lack of women's voices who are rarely, if ever, asked what they want or need; who are often given medication they do not want; and who are rarely asked if the treatment they have been given actually worked.

Why is it that the importance of women and their role in carrying, birthing and raising the next generation is so seriously negated in many cultures? Why has it taken so long for society to finally realise that fathers, partners and adoptive parents also feel huge strain through this process too? Yet, humanity is dependent upon the next generation for its future survival.

Humans do not seem to be good at learning from past mistakes. It is easier to keep our heads in the sand and act as if nothing is wrong. Yet, something is seriously wrong. More children today are experiencing anxiety and depression than ever before. The diagnosis of neurodivergency is exploding, and mental health is declining. The COVID-19 pandemic has also compounded the difficulties, as has the fear of environmental catastrophe. Fundamentally, we are ignoring the research showing the impact of struggles in pre-conception and in utero on the infant. When experiencing birth, women often talk of feeling ignored and of having little choice. Post birth, parents who struggle to raise their children in societies where life is so expensive that a single wage is not enough to keep mouths fed, bills paid and a roof over the family's head feel ignored and neglected. These children are our future. They need our investment, both in money but more importantly in love and time.

It is not all bleak. When I began this work, nobody was particularly interested in what I did, it was considered pretty niche. However, slowly, I am perceiving a subtle shift. More partners now come to learn how they can help when their partner has severe maternal mental illness. More couples come with conception, infertility and difficulties with termination for medical reasons. More fathers are asking what their role is, rather than taking it for granted that it is the woman's role to raise the children and run the house (as well as hold down a full-time job or career). More therapists are coming for training and asking how to get into this work. More groups are being set up offering therapeutic support and validation. In the UK, the Duchess of Cambridge, for example, has set up the 'First 1,000 days' project, drawing attention to this period as the fundamental time when brain development is at its fastest and greatest level. Research is beginning to find out and learn about what causes miscarriage and infertility. And in the UK and elsewhere health services are having to do U-turns: from closing down the vast majority of MBUs, and cutting perinatal services, to finally recognising the considerable need and the detrimental result of closing down services. These are the seeds of change. However, this is not cause for passivity or complacency. The black hole is vast.

This book is about passion, love and nurture. It is also about listening and truly hearing women's experience. As Ernest Hemingway says – 'when people talk, listen completely. Most people never listen' (1949, p. 90). This book is also about experience – what it was like for me to work with the many women, men and partners I have seen over the years since I walked into that MBU, and then chose to specialise in private practice in maternal mental illness and trauma.

However, this book is only one-half of the story. My practice is in two interwoven parts – maternal and paternal mental health: helping the parents to feel well enough to bond, develop and flourish with their children – and the other part, when it goes wrong: the consequences of neglect and dysfunctional parenting, working with developmental trauma, the earliest and most devastating trauma. These intertwine, informing one another, and helping me to form a picture of the environment from pre-conception through to adulthood.

Let me use Eric Berne's brilliant metaphor of the stack of pennies (Berne, 1975 [1961]) to represent a person's personality, from pre-conception through to adulthood. Berne suggested that any emotional or physical trauma would be shown as a penny misaligned with the stack, compromising the stacks stability, and risking the (psychological) stack toppling over. The earlier the relational trauma, the more fundamental the impact of that trauma on the child's psychological and emotional development and the greater the risk to the child's future psychopathology. Focusing on maternal mental illness helps a parent to recognise (relationally, emotionally, psychologically and bodily) the impact of those earliest traumas on their child (the relational ruptures) and gives the opportunity to gently re-align the impacted metaphorical penny in their child's developing psyche (the relational repair), because 'the lower down the warped coin is, the greater its effect on the ultimate stability' (Berne, 1975 [1961], p. 54).

In writing this book, my aim is to help psychotherapists begin to understand that they can fundamentally help a person to change their life decisions, to choose a new pathway and to effect change that has longevity. Relational psychotherapy offers a way to treat the cause of mental illness. If it is done well, with an ethical stance and flexibility on the part of the therapist with a focus on the uniqueness of each person's illness, we can effect change that leads to a lifetime of improved mental wellness. We are not broken – we may be battered and bruised by our traumas – yet the neuroplasticity of our brains and the continual progress of human development in each and every one of us allows the possibility of fundamental, psychological change.

This book is a beginning and I hope it will plant a seed for you all to nurture and grow. It is not and never will be perfect or complete, much as parenthood is never perfect and complete. Writing it has been messy and chaotic. Sometimes it has felt like paints, Play-Doh and LEGO have been scattered all over my floor ready for me to painfully step on it or frustratingly tread it into the carpet. At other times, no doubt those around me have felt like the book I was nurturing and developing was my own newborn baby. I cannot stop as I absolutely love my work. My clients shock me, teach me, help me to be creative and inspire me. I hope I never stop learning from them. This book is for each and every one of them; you all know who you are, with my love. It is also for every parent in the world, no matter who you are, or where you live. You are unique and special. You deserve to be listened to, and helped, in whatever way you need. Yes, it absolutely does take a village to raise a child. It also takes a healthy world environment to continue to raise a healthy human race.

References

Berne, E. (1975). *Transactional Analysis in Psychotherapy: A Systematic Individual and Social Psychiatry*. London: Souvenir Press. (Original work published 1961.)

Hemingway, E. (1949). Letter of advice to a young writer, reported in Malcolm Cowley, 'Mister papa'. *LIFE Magazine*, Jan 10, 26(2), p. 90.

Stern, D., Bruschweiler-Stern, N., and Freeland, A. (1998). *The Birth of a Mother*. New York: Basic Books

Acknowledgements

There are so many people who have encouraged me, inspired me and helped me in my journey towards writing this book. Firstly, I would like to thank my husband, Andy, for being an absolutely fantastic husband during the lengthy process of writing, and for his tireless ability to cope with my whirring brain and the inevitable middle of the night writing. I would like to thank my children, David, Anna-Cristina and Georgina, for their patience and understanding. Inevitably, the book was my newest baby, and took a great deal of my focus. I would also like to wholeheartedly thank Debs Hill for reading the entire book and applying her superb editing skills. I could not have done this without you, Debs.

Three men encouraged me to go forward to write about this subject – Mark Widdowson, Professor John McLeod and Giles Barrow, and I owe a great deal to all three. In particular, Mark has been a tireless supporter from the day I turned up in his office as his newest PhD student and he has never stopped encouraging and supporting me since then. I will be eternally grateful for all his guidance and sound advice, as well as his ability to trust me in my creative process. All three men have encouraged me to take this forward, to write more, to explore more, to speak up for all those women who cannot. I am indebted to them all and I will continue researching and writing.

Particular friends and colleagues have been wonderfully generous in reading and critiquing each and every chapter: Lou Walker, Janice Butler, Sarah Hobhouse, Daphne Winning, Marie-Louise Johnson, Wilf Hashimi, Marion Umney, Sue Eusden, Holly Radford, Birgitta Heiller, Rachel Cook, Dr Jane Hanley and Hayley Manning. You have all helped me craft this book into something readable and hopefully useful. To all my other friends who lost me for a year or so, sorry, I am back now.

To my supervisees and trainees who have continued to challenge my thinking, my creativity and my conceptualisation of my type of treatment – thank you. You have made me a better trainer and supervisor. And to Cathy Lasher, I thank you for advocating for me for time to write; I so appreciate it.

To the next generation of therapists who are coming along behind, I hope to inspire you to live your passion and dream. No matter how many people try and thwart you on the way, no matter how many brick walls you feel you are up against, you will get there, you will do it and you will achieve your dream.

To the international transactional analysis community – I am so proud to be a part of you, for the rigour of training and examining, for the depth and breadth of theory, which is phenomenal and for the knowledge and encouragement from so many of the truly great and influential people in the community – Charlotte Sills, Bill Cornell, Helena Hargaden, Adrienne Lee, Trudi Newton, Robin Fryer, Biljana van Rijn, Karen Minikin, Leilani Mitchell and Helen Rowland, to name just a few of this astonishing and growing community. For me, TA changed my life and challenged me hard, and this has made me the best therapist I could ever be. Thank you everyone.

And finally, to my clients – to you all I owe you the most. I am indebted to you for sticking with the process and for trusting me. To those of you who have agreed to be a part of my research each and every one of you has taught me everything I know. You are unique and it has been an honour to be a part of your treatment journey. You deserve to feel as good as you can, to mother in your own special way. Go well.

All of the client vignettes in this book are derived from my clinical and teaching experience. In order to keep privacy, I have substantially altered names and circumstances. I have also amalgamated many stories so that they are unrecognisable. However, there are two clients whose stories I have not altered substantially and who have given full permission to be included in this book: I thank you 'Laura' for your generous agreement to let me share your creative object and your experience of postpartum psychosis; and Ania, I thank you for agreeing to me sharing your experience of needle phobia and how it led onto you experiencing tokophobia.

Permissions

The following extract was originally published elsewhere:

Part I
Hear Us Speak

1 Transitions

There is a long-standing and nostalgic perception that motherhood is a rosy, wonderful time, full of scented unicorns and fluorescent sparkling bubbles, when the mother is simply overjoyed with her baby, bonding instantly immediately after birth. This perception is perpetuated socially, culturally and inter-generationally, and assumes that women instinctively know how to give birth, how to breastfeed and how to care for their infant. The perception even seems to assume that as childbirth is a natural process, it comes with little pain.

But what if a woman struggles with any of these things, and research suggests that a significant silent cohort does? She is met with disbelief and her experience is discounted, or dismissed.

The myths of motherhood seem entrenched in every part of Western society, particularly on social media and in advertisements, within family, friends and neighbours whose response to a mother with mental illness can often be silencing and shaming. Culture continues to be reluctant to let go of these myths, continuing to situate motherhood in a binary position as either a time of bliss, everything wonderful, glossy and glorious, or alternatively, positioning the mother as bad and blamed for everything that happens in her child's life. The reality is that many women find the transitions from conception, through pregnancy and the postnatal period riddled with anxiety and stress, fear, guilt and shame, and a time when they feel constantly under pressure to be the 'perfect mother'.

Why are so many women unwell during pregnancy and postnatally? Unfortunately, this is a difficult question to answer as there is no real consensus on the causes. Hypotheses range from it being a physical disorder, caused by hormone fluctuations, to being a sociological condition, caused by high expectations from society and mothers themselves. It has also been viewed as a malfunction of mental processes caused by the social difficulties a mother is experiencing. Whatever the cause, and these may be numerous and specific to the mother involved, we need to come to terms with the fact that many women are unwell and struggle at some point in their transition to becoming a mother.

Understanding why women become mentally ill around childbirth is important. Yet this is not a book about why. This book focuses on how we can

DOI: 10.4324/9781003154891-2

help women and any parent in their time of struggle. When a woman, man or couple come through my door for therapy, my focus is on 'what do you need', 'how can I help you', 'how can I enable you so you can begin to make sense of what is happening and navigate a pathway through your distress'?

This book is not a protocol nor is it a manualised treatment. Relational psychotherapy cannot be manualised. Relational psychotherapy changes the philosophical focus of psychotherapeutic change from the belief that it occurs from the development of insight, to one focused on conscious and unconscious developmental and relational difficulties, explored and addressed within the therapeutic relationship. This book does not and can never offer all the answers, because every new client I see will have mental illness specific to them. What this book does give the reader is all the elements I have found to be important to know and use when working with maternal mental illness. Nor is this book an exhaustive exploration of all the research. It is not a book for academics. It is a guide for clinicians. I have included as much research as I think is necessary. In each of the chapters, there will be enough resources to explore and expand knowledge. Research is updated all the time, so whatever is in the book will almost certainly be out of date as soon as it is published.

I am not a medical doctor, but a psychotherapist. I have a profound belief in listening to and hearing my client's distress at the deepest level, then working collaboratively, through transparency and open communication, to find a way forward. Fundamentally, it is always a way that my client wants to take, and is never a pathway that I choose, unilaterally, for my client. For me, mutuality and interconnectedness form an important part of this relational dyad. As does equality. Power is inherent in the relationship because I am the therapist and, therefore, I may be seen as the 'expert', sitting in the chair of power. My client may come to therapy feeling acutely not OK in herself, in her relationships, in society, but with a sense that others are indeed OK. Immediately, she will feel in the one-down position, so my focus is on this asymmetry of power. My clients often say they feel their mental illness puts them on the margins of society. Silence continues the marginalisation because silence stops women from speaking up and speaking out. If they do not speak up and speak out, they do not get help. Oppression is a large part of this illness.

The transformation to motherhood

Daniel Stern's research shows that when a woman transitions from being someone's child into being someone's mother, something fundamental happens. Motherhood changes that woman. From the moment of conception, during pregnancy, through the birth process and afterwards, a woman transforms into someone she was not before. This transformation happens through both hormones and experience. Of course, she has never been pregnant before, she has not given birth or ever been a mother. This change begins gradually but eventually she will 'operate from an entirely new mindset' (Stern, Bruschweiler-Stern & Freeland, 1998, p. 5). This transition into a mother is important for species survival and also due to the responsibility of raising a child, which a woman needs to step up to. Her new mindset will be filled with structure and thought around the infant, changing every aspect of her prior relationships, shifting her focus onto her infant. Both physically and mentally there will be a new life path, one that is centred around the infant, learning constantly how to cope with new tasks, how to feed, look after, cope with an infant, when to be concerned, when not to be, when to call a doctor and when to calm down.

The change is transformative; it can be nothing else. For some, it may be full of joy. For others, it may be riddled with chores, fear, lack of self-esteem, anxiety and any number of other negative emotions, such as guilt and shame, upsetting the woman's mental health considerably. For some, this new mindset will be there forever, dominating the woman and making her feel 'less than'. Others may find their negative emotions subside once they begin to feel more in control and able, allowing her to put new and different things into that central position. One of these things may be work, due to a financial need to go back to work or a desire to get back to a familiar structure. This subsidence of the mindset will not stop the mother stepping in immediately if their child needs it, due to ill-health, danger or difficulties. For the majority of mothers, even when their child is an adult and has no longer lived with them for many years, this feeling of responsibility for the child – even if the child is a successful adult in their own right – never goes away, and that mother–infant bond is lit again.

This book is not about when the transformation goes well, and bonding takes place. It is about how to help those women who struggle with this transformation and who find themselves in a place where they are unable to enjoy being a parent. Everyone at some stage or another will struggle with becoming and being a parent. It is not for nothing that there is an old saying that parenting is the hardest job in the world. It can push a person to the very edges of emotion and experience. This may be due to a plethora of reasons such as experiencing a poor childhood with little in the way of role models, leaving a person with few resources to use. It could be due to lack of stability in a relationship, ending with becoming a single parent with its huge challenges. It also is most likely due to prior mental health conditions which seem to be stirred again, almost certainly due to a mixture of responsibilities, hormone surges, emotional surges, lack of sleep and exhaustion after the birth process.

What I hope to convey to you as the reader is that none of this is abnormal and that there is always hope. Most women arrive at my door thinking they are 'unfixable', as if there is something profoundly wrong with them. No there is not. The hill to climb, out of these feelings and emotions, can seem steep. But it is not insurmountable. However, it needs to be climbed with others, so they can help when the going gets tough. It is difficult, if not almost impossible to do on your own.

Motherhood is a relational process. From conception, and for some, even prior to conception, a mother is in a relationship with her fetus and this relationship continues throughout life until there is a rupture. Therefore, it makes sense to me to treat it within a relational paradigm, in particular using relational psychotherapy. Maternity care is also relational, yet this is not always the experience my clients have received. Of course, my clients are those who are struggling within the motherhood timeframe, and so it may be perceived that I am overly influenced by negative experiences. However, I am a mother, and I have many friends who are mothers, and I am worried by what I read and hear about obstetric care. But what I find most baffling is the lack of empathy, compassion and interest afforded to aftercare. Newborn babies are totally helpless, reliant on those caring for them for 100% of their needs. Babies do not come with a manual. Yet mothers are expected to know instinctively how to look after them, how to address their needs, how to cope, with little or no help. Culturally, within the Western world, motherhood is portrayed as this wonderful, easy and natural experience. For those who find it so, they are the lucky few. For the rest, there continues to be a culture of silence, with many women suffering in silence. My concern is for these women and their children. Their children are a fundamental part of this damaging system and are affected down the line, as I discuss in Chapter 2. Yet, their mothers are given little or no psychological support when they need it most, within those first few years of pregnancy and after birth. It is implausible that in the 21st century we still do not train psychotherapists to treat maternal mental illness. Instead, we rely on pharmacologically focused medical practitioners who give out pills, some with interesting research results when used in pregnancy and during breastfeeding, as a way for a woman to try and control her symptoms (see Chapter 17 for a more detailed review on conventional treatment).

There has to be a better way forward, a more inclusive, compassionate and empathetic way to help women bring up our future generations so that we do not condemn them to the same issues their parents experienced. Too much money is being spent on the aftermath of a poor maternal attachment environment. Would that money not be better spent if it was focused on the beginning of a child's life, rather than mopping up the deleterious effects, years after the event? We need to focus as a society, on the long term: on our future and our children. We need to offer our children the best start in life that is possible. To do that, we need to focus our attention towards truly helping women with childbirth and parenthood, not simply accepting what is currently the norm. I hear too many women talk about their distress, the gynaecological violence they experience after having a miscarriage for example, the lack of time to speak or to be heard, the lack of care they are offered and the lack of answers when there is a difficulty with conception or in pregnancy.

Having spent the large part of my professional work specialising in this area, I strongly believe that all psychotherapists, and any other health professionals, need to learn about this area, and how they may help. Motherhood, father-hood and raising children are a fundamental part of so many lives. We teach about working with anxiety, stress and depression, yet for some reason, we don't look at the causes of these conditions. Maybe it is just me, but it would seem that society, the government, organisations, psychotherapy training institutes, the medical systems and culture all seem to have their heads buried in the sand.

Maternal mental illness is common and has huge consequences for the mother, the infant, the wider family and the economy. Yet it is rarely talked about and often goes undiagnosed and untreated. There is little written about it, other than a few books narrating first-hand experiences. Although there is some academic research, that research is not widely disseminated. Women and professionals alike are often confused by the symptoms and the lack of written material, which leads to misunderstanding and misdiagnosis and per-petuates the silence about their condition.

Women remain silent for many reasons: guilt about not living up to the 'perfect' mother portrayed in books and on social media; shame about their perceived inability, weakness or laziness as a mother; fear of being judged for not coping (because all other mothers do cope, don't they?); fear of the reper-cussions of admitting their struggle – will they have a black mark against them from their doctor or health visitor, will they then be at risk of having the baby removed by social services?; fear of the damage they are doing to their child. The list is endless. However, there is one thing very clear about motherhood in Western society: mothers are judged and most often that judgement is negative. Mothers are often perceived to be the bad person, the one that damages their child, the one who didn't care enough, the one who didn't meet their child's needs, the reason why a child becomes seen as 'delinquent'. Mothers get a pretty bad press. Often, they can feel damned if they do and damned if they don't, another bind to add to the many that women find themselves in. Motherhood is shown in such a binary fashion in Western society – either you are the 'good' mother, the fairytale princess mother who attends absolutely and utterly to your child's needs. Or you are a bad mother – a wicked witch who neglects and abuses your baby, causing that infant to grow up with lifelong consequences. The media and society play a huge part in perpetuating this binary system.

And there begins the bind for women. The unrealistic portrayal of what motherhood 'should' be like can lead to a sense of deep discontentment, guilt and huge shame. It can also lead to an 'is this it?' moment of realisation, that yes, this is actually it. Sleep deprivation, heightened emotions, extreme fatigue, a relentless feeling of demands on your time, with not enough time for anything, least of all a hot cup of tea. And a sense of will you ever get any of your life back?

So, bringing up a child is difficult at the best of times and excruciating at the worst, when a woman experiences physical or mental illness. The bind then becomes about who is more important: infant or mother? Many women are a little shocked with the process of a hospital birth and can feel that the baby is more important than they are. This question of who is most important continues into mental illness post birth. Is it better for a woman to take anti-depressants or other medication and continue to breastfeed, or should the woman stop breastfeeding? Or should the woman try and struggle on without the medication because she believes her baby's well-being is more important? Women who are unwell on the whole still care for their babies to the best of their ability, even if that ability is severely restricted. Yet women are continuously bound up in advice of 'what is best'. But best for whom?

Breastfeeding is a case in point, as some women will struggle for weeks or months trying desperately to breastfeed because they feel they 'should' be able to, or 'should' know how to because they are female, regardless of how it is making them feel. Rarely are women told that for some it simply does not work no matter how much you try. Yes 'breast is best' is an important message, until it becomes a guilt trip to send a woman on because she is finding it unbearably difficult or if her baby does not thrive. And let's remember that some women are physically unable to breastfeed at all.

No matter who we are, a mother, a father, a partner, a care giver or an adoptive parent, an infant will change our life. And no matter how realistic we are in pregnancy or prior to conception, we do not know how life will change; no-one knows. We may have an idea, but it is rarely the same as the reality.

Perhaps part of the problem stems from our modern way of living in the 21st century. In the Western world, families have become more disparate and there may no longer be the extended family or friends to help to raise the infant together. There is an African proverb which say it takes a village to raise a child (attributed to different African cultures and then used by Hilary Clinton in her 1996 book *It Takes a Village: And Other Lessons Children Teach Us*). However, these days many cultures do not fit this village metaphor anymore and parenting often then becomes quite a solitary role for mothers and parents.

So, what is my aim in writing this book? I have already talked about beginning to fill the yawning, enormous gap that exists for psychotherapists, counsellors and health practitioners who are not taught about this condition, nor given guidance on suitable treatment options to offer. I do not have all the answers, nobody does. However, I do know that women often tell me they would very much prefer psychological therapy in preference to drug treatment. However, without a thorough training and in-depth knowledge how can we help these women to the best of our professional ability? I also want to draw attention to the complexity of the ethical dilemmas involved in maternal mental illness. What I have discovered over the years is a dizzying array of questions and options, from pre-conception through to raising the child. Also, I want to highlight what it is like for a woman who is neurodivergent to raise a child that may also be neurodivergent, yet may be neurotypical too.

There is virtually nothing written about neurodivergence, motherhood and psychotherapy, and consequently, recent research shows that the vast majority of psychotherapists have little knowledge and feel ill-equipped to offer treatment (see Chapter 15 for a more in-depth exploration).

However, I believe this book goes further than informing professional practice. It may also be useful for women experiencing this condition, any family members who are impacted and also healthcare workers such as doctors, midwives and health visitors. I aim to try to give a solid understanding of the nature and complexity of this illness.

There are also some crucial elements about treatment that do not seem to be acknowledged within the medical world which I believe are vitally important, such as the specificity of the illness. By that I mean that for each woman, mental illness is often unique. They may have similar symptoms to others, but the way in which they experience those symptoms can be very different. As a professional offering treatment this is vital knowledge. I need to help the person in front of me and address their own uniqueness. I could offer a generic, 12 step manualised treatment, that might or might not work for the person in front of me, but I don't. I want women to use their experience of treatment as a way forward to have a lifetime reduction in their mental ill health. People have history, and often it is this history that gives this illness its clout. For many years it has been well known that people with an underlying history of mental illness may be more susceptible to illness within pregnancy and the postnatal period. Despite many hypotheses, there are no useful conclusions as to why this might be. In the years I have spent treating women and partners, I have found that for many clients there is a mix of elements that come together to form something like a catastrophic time bomb which explodes either within pregnancy or shortly after childbirth.

But maternal mental illness is also so much more than this catastrophic time bomb. There are many other aspects that need to be included and that I have tried to cover in the book. In my Ph.D. research, I was shocked to find that nearly every single research project excluded women with postpartum psychosis. I could not believe that women with this hugely distressing condition were being excluded. This felt very much a parallel to what happens to them in society when they have this condition, as they say they often feel very much excluded. This exclusion is likely to be due to the need to get research through an ethical panel, which can be difficult due to the concern about harm to the participants, particularly when researching mental illness. I was determined to include postpartum psychosis in my research, because I see the aftermath of it in my clinical practice. Psychosis is rare, but to those women and their families who have it, it can be utterly devastating. Leaving them out helps no-one with their understanding. I also have a chapter on maternal trauma, as although birth trauma is now the focus of more research, there is not enough spoken about the other different traumas and how these can have an impact in the perinatal period, such as tokophobia, hyperemesis gravidarum, miscarriage, infertility, termination for medical reasons, still-birth and neonatal loss and rape and sexual abuse.

We must remember that maternal mental illness is treatable. For the woman to move towards a lifetime reduction in mental illness, however, it is not enough to solely prescribe medication. My focus, in psychotherapy, is on addressing the cause of their illness, not through symptomatic relief, although symptoms do subside usually quite quickly. I am not against pre-scription medication, as it can be useful as a short-term gap when women are very distressed. To get long-term, sustainable results, it is often necessary to use long-term therapy. This may be difficult in a medical system which is always challenged with funding, although group therapy, when carefully thought through and managed, works just as effectively. However, at the outset one-to-one can often be more effective, because many women feel too much shame and guilt to be part of a group.

Quite often a woman can be frightened of a subsequent pregnancy. I have seen women who experienced mental illness in their first pregnancy and received no treatment through their doctor. I have also seen clients return because they are convinced it will all begin again with the next pregnancy. It often does not begin again. And it is absolutely OK for those women to seek reassurance from me for their fear. Once they begin to realise it is not com-ing back, often that is enough for them to forge out on their own, without needing my help anymore.

Most of the women who come to my therapy room had no idea that there was any treatment available, until they googled and found me. I am not someone special at all, I simply realised that there was no treatment on offer. Here are the key things I found which I think clinicians need to know and understand:

- Most people continue to call any kind of mental illness in motherhood 'postnatal depression'. This is extremely unhelpful to pregnant women and also to those who do not feel depressed, but feel distressed, anxious, overwhelmed, frightened, guilty, ashamed and as if they are going mad. I explore this more later in this chapter.
- Maternal mental illness covers a wide variety of different elements: dis-tress, anxiety, grief, trauma and distress, but also infertility, psychosis, miscarriage, IVF and indeed whatever else a client brings that has caused her to feel distressed by motherhood.
- Women who are unwell often have had symptoms in pregnancy but tried desperately to keep a lid on it and not mention it in the hopes that once the baby came that would be enough for them to get better.
- The woman will often struggle on, feeling dreadful, trying to keep on top of all she has to do, often becoming more and more unwell, until crisis point, at which she is unable to continue to function and is often extremely unwell.
- Men, partners and adoptive parents can be unwell too.

- Elements from the past can seriously impact the pregnancy and birth, such as sexual assault or childhood sexual abuse, trauma and a difficult and traumatic childhood.
- Many more women experience symptoms than we think.
- Without treatment, this illness can continue for a lifetime.

Semantics

Before I go much further, I would like to say a few things about semantics. Throughout this book, I will use the term woman/women. Men, partners in single sex relationships and adoptive parents can also experience mental illness in their transition to becoming parents. However, because it is women who make up the vast majority of cases, I have chosen to use these terms only. As yet though, being pregnant and giving birth are still a totally female domain and may be the one area left within the world where gender stereotyping is still acceptable. Please forgive me!

I use the term perinatal throughout the book. The term perinatal has different ways to define it – the National Health Service (NHS) in the UK defines it as simply pregnancy through to 1-year post birth (NHS England, 2018). Several medical textbooks, particularly those published in USA also use the term peripartum instead of perinatal. The Diagnostic and Statistical Manual (DSM-5) seems to define peripartum as pregnancy and 4 weeks following delivery (APA, 2013, p. 152). Medical textbooks may also dispute the time I have given to post birth and insist that the perinatal period ends around 6 weeks post birth. However, clinically, and within this book I use maternal and perinatal as catch-all words. I have seen women who are several years post birth and I will still use the term perinatal mental illness, if the symptoms began in pregnancy or postnatally. In fact, I have even seen a woman about 20 years post birth, who had never received treatment. Her symptoms of illness bore a huge familiarity to those I see in women who have just given birth. She continued to be distressed about her birth experience and struggled with her mood even after such a long period of time had elapsed.

Throughout the book I use the term maternal mental illness, which I prefer to perinatal. I use it purposefully, because it encapsulates not only all the different experiences women have, but the term is purposefully not time specific, as I believe there is no real time limit to this condition. When people talk about maternal mental illness, they most often call it 'postnatal depression'. Unfortunately, in some countries, there seems to be a difficulty in acknowledging that postnatal depression is only a small part of the problems. Even in 2019, the US Preventive Services Task Force still continued to refer to perinatal depression and issued draft recommendations about prevention of perinatal depression. This term is used culturally in the Western world as a 'catch all' for anything relating to mental illness in motherhood. Yet, I have two main difficulties with it. Firstly, calling it depression is not accurate. Yes, some women definitely do display signs of depression. Yet, the majority of women I see tend to be more anxious and stressed than depressed. Many seem to be in a state of hyperarousal, with an overwhelming sense of distress and a need to be calmed and soothed, something that they seem unable to do for themselves. Extreme fear is also a common feature. They are on alert for anything and everything that heightens their stress and distress. Many women find it difficult to voice this fear, almost certainly due to a variety of reasons such as fear that they might have their baby removed from their care, or a sense that there is something fundamentally wrong with them because they do not fit the cultural stereotype of the happy, contented mother they feel they should be.

Mode of practice

I know that whatever I write will be judged by some to be incorrect. I write this book from the position of a psychotherapist treating women with maternal mental illness, sitting at what I believe is the cutting edge of treatment; it is my life and my career. Many of the women and partners I see have come to me because they have received little or no help from an inadequately trained medical profession and are at a loss as to how to gain any help at all.

I also know that I come from a place of bias, as do all of us. I am a mother of three grown-up children, so I come from a place of empathy and understanding. I know what it feels like to go through some of the things that are talked about in this book. This book is not about me, however. It is about my clients, and the rich and diverse lessons they have taught me about motherhood, mental illness, distress and the number of difficulties they have brought. The most important thing in psychotherapy is to see the person in front of you as a human being, offering empathy and understanding, being curious about their experience and never ever trying to fit their experience into a box of similar experiences. Each of my clients is unique. Maternal mental illness is also unique. Also, no matter how hard society tries to box it up into symptoms and diagnoses, I refuse to call my area of expertise maternal mental *health*. This would portray something positive, yet those I see are not healthy, they are unwell. So, calling it 'health' feels like I am discounting just how unwell they actually are. However, calling it illness, I also find difficult. Is this an illness? What is an illness? These women do not have a disease. Above all, they are distressed.

If a woman tells me she is extremely unwell, I know for her she is scared and feels extremely unwell. I don't need to decide that I know better than her. I am not the expert in her. She is. Similarly, when I see women post birth who are struggling with an infant that won't sleep or won't feed, I am not judging her or thinking about her incapacity to fulfil those tasks. I am hearing that her infant is distressed and that she is also distressed. My aim is to help both her and her infant gain a place of calm and tranquillity, so that they can both get back to simply being – mother and infant.

Many of my clients tell me they have struggled to gain any kind of treatment for their distress, so have turned towards the private sector for help. I use Transactional Analysis (TA) psychotherapy in my work with my clients, and

I find it a useful form of treatment. For me, there are elements in TA theory, particularly within relational TA theory (Cornell & Hargaden, 2005; Fowlie & Sills, 2011; Hargaden & Sills, 2002), as well as co-creative theory (Summers & Tudor, 2000) and Transgenerational Scripting (Noriega Gayol, 2004), that are particularly useful and valuable in increasing a women's understanding of her distress. Relational TA theory also highlights the importance and value of a mother's bond with her infant, the importance of conscious and non-conscious patterns of relating and experience, the importance of the relationship, its co-creative nature, and the importance of the mother/father/caregiver in modelling behaviour both explicitly and implicitly within the infant/parent bond.

However, this book is not focused only at TA psychotherapists. I have written it in a way that I hope will speak to any psychotherapist. This book is about inclusivity. Every psychotherapist can work with maternal mental illness. For me, I find relational psychotherapy works the best. That is why this book focuses on the relationship, rather than being modality specific. I continue to research TA because I find it to be a powerful and effective model of therapy for this condition.

Plan of the book

This book is in two parts – the first part, I have called 'Hear us speak'. This part is about listening to women's voices, and to the information we already know: from statistics about prevalence and cost in Chapter 2, the historical aspects in Chapter 3, the common conditions in Chapter 4, maternal trauma in Chapter 5, postpartum psychosis in Chapter 6, narratives of maternal mental illness in Chapter 7 and finishing with barriers to treatment in Chapter 8. We need to *hear* what these women are saying. All of these chapters help to build a picture of the complexity of this illness, how it has been present, spoken and written about for millennia, yet even now no-one knows exactly what it is. They highlight the depth and breadth of this illness which is vast, and which I emphasise in Chapters 4–7. Finally, I include the many and enduring barriers to treatment which continually thwart women in receiving anything other than medication, which women consistently say they don't want.

The second part of the book is called 'Listening beyond words' and it is, in essence, about treatment – how relational psychotherapy not only treats the woman's mental illness, the cause of which that may have been lurking for many years, it is the fundamental positive impact this also has on her child and family that are of added bonus. We are not, and never will be, only treating the woman – we are actually treating an entire family system, because if the woman is functioning well in relationship to her intimate others: partners, children, friends and family, then everyone benefits. I use the phrase 'listening beyond words' because a great deal of the techniques I use are based on visual clues – movements, gestures and behaviours, but also from verb sequencing, reverie, intuition and paralinguistics, offering me a bodily felt sense which allows me to focus on our transferential relationship.

Treatment is developmental and evolves with the therapeutic relationship. It is similar to the needs of an infant in the first years of life, which I highlight in Chapters 12 and 13: beginning by addressing the distress, then moving onto particular elements which are vital, such as attachment, attunement, implicit relational knowing and affect regulation. Part II begins with the arguments for and critique against relational psychotherapy in Chapter 9; the different ethical dilemmas we might see in Chapter 10; why it is so important to treat the cause rather than simply focus on symptomatic relief in Chapter 11; the fundamental need all humans have – the ability to regulate our own affect in Chapter 12; the therapeutic role in Chapter 13; using creativity with this client group in Chapter 14; neurodivergency and motherhood in Chapter 15; working with partners and couples in Chapter 16; and finishing with a brief look at conventional (drug) treatment in Chapter 17. The book ends with a short, aspirational chapter on how relational psychotherapy can help to bring about a lifetime reduction in mental illness.

You may wonder, at this point, why I have left out fathers and partners. They are threaded through this book. However, fathers and partners actually warrant their own book. The research into their mental illness in the transition to parenthood is burgeoning and finally there is now recognition that adoptive parents struggle with mental illness too. I cannot do fathers and partners justice in only one chapter, and word count meant it would have been a meagre chapter at that, although I thought carefully about leaving them out. Fathers, partners and adoptive parents deserve a great deal more. Frankly, the impact on the entire family system from parental mental illness needs a spotlight shone on it. We cannot continue ignoring what stares us in the face. If we plough resources into parenthood, we benefit the entire family, not just the parents. This is money well spent.

References

APA (2013). *Diagnostic and Statistical Manual of Mental Disorders*, Fifth Edition. Arlington, VA.: American Psychiatric Association.

Cornell, W.F., and Hargaden, H. (Eds) (2005). *From Transactions to Relations: the Emergence of a Relational Tradition in Transactional Analysis*. Chadlington, UK: Haddon Press.

Fowlie, H., and Sills, C. (2011). *Relational Transactional Analysis: Principles in Practice*. London: Karnac.

Hargaden, H., and Sills, C. (2002). *Transactional Analysis: A Relational Perspective*. Hove, UK: Brunner-Routledge.

NHS England (2018). *The Perinatal Mental Health Care Pathways*. NHS England.

Noriega Gayol, G. (2004). Codependence: A transgenerational script. *Transactional Analysis Journal*, 34(4), p. 312–322.

Stern, D.N., Bruschweiler-Stern, N., and Freeland, A. (1998). *The Birth of a Mother. How the Motherhood Experience Changes You Forever*. New York: Basic Books.

Summers, G., and Tudor, K. (2000). Co-creative transactional analysis. *Transactional Analysis Journal*, 30(10), p. 23–40.

2   A Silent Problem

Many women experience mental illness at some point from conception to post birth. Maternal mental illness is not new and has been known about for hundreds of years, possibly even from the time of Hippocrates. Yet still today, there is no real agreement on why it occurs, what the effects are on the woman, the infant or the family, nor what the correct treatment actually is, if indeed there is treatment offered. For many, the illness continues to be misdiagnosed and mistreated.

The sobering fact is that this illness is common and it has a wide-reaching impact on the mother, the child, the family and the economy, and is the leading cause of maternal mortality in pregnancy (Howard & Khalifeh, 2020; Howard et al., 2014). In the most recent Mothers and Babies: Reducing Risk through Audits and Confidential Enquiries (MBRRACE) Report (Knight et al., 2019) maternal suicide is still the second leading direct cause of death during pregnancy and within the first 42 days post birth in the UK. Research has consistently focused mainly on the postnatal period and particularly on depression. Even relatively recently, mental health issues have tended to be diagnosed as either the baby blues, postnatal depression or postpartum psychosis, all of which were deemed to occur only in the postnatal period. Focussing on postnatal depression is probably due to the lack of agreement between health professionals on the pathogenesis of mental illness within this period. However, in the past 10 years, the term 'perinatal' has been more widely used, reflecting a shift in comprehension of the depth and breadth of this condition. The term 'peripartum', the term more widely used in North America, has even been adopted within the Diagnostic and Statistical Manual of Mental Health (DSM-V) (APA, 2013), and this is because research shows that 50% of diagnoses of postnatal depression actually begin within the antenatal period (APA, 2013, p. 152).

There are so many differing hypotheses or theories about maternal mental illness as well as continuing philosophical debates about how to most effectively diagnose and treat this illness. This is not helped by the multitude of myths around pregnancy, childbirth and parenthood, which continue to be perpetuated societally and culturally. Myths such as breastfeeding will stop the onset of mental illness, that feeding needs to be done on a four-hourly

DOI: 10.4324/9781003154891-3

schedule and feeding on demand produces a needy child. These myths and many others only serve to place women under the strain of guilt (they can never reach the position of 'perfect' mother) and the burden of responsibility of caring for the child and trying to hold down a job to keep the family afloat financially, in this ever more expensive world we live in. There is also something about motherhood becoming a performance (and has been since the beginning of the 20th century). There are numerous manuals explaining how to do it 'successfully', which quite often contradict each other, about the need for empathy and compassion, with the advent of the 24-hour mother. Yet knowledge is still missing, and the refrain 'why did no-one ever tell me', which was even to become the title of Hollie McNish's book *Nobody told me*, is still prevalent. We are expected to know what our child needs and to respond to them accordingly, tolerating the difficult behaviour; to educate the child (on top of it being educated at school); to give the child its freedom to explore and experience; to generate fun for the child and to stimulate it continuously. There is increased pressure to perform as a mother, yet with less and less resources of time, money, and help. At the same time, mothering has become one of the most difficult and attacked roles in society, with mothers being the problem and the solution to all their child's ills. Mother is accused of emasculating her sons and suffocating her daughters (Thurer, 1994); she is told to love her children unconditionally but not love them too much in case the child becomes too needy and time-consuming. She must not be neglectful, yet is told to put her child into child-care, allowing someone else to raise her child, whilst she goes out to work to help pay the mortgage or put food on the table. All-in-all a mother's lot is confusing, difficult, guilt-ridden, shameful, stressful, anxiety-inducing and isolating. Add to this the difficulty in conception, particularly in the Western world with a declining fertility rate and many more couples struggling to conceive naturally and having to resort to IVF or to artificial reproductive techniques (ART). Then add the difficulties of miscarriage, with levels much higher than realised, the possibility of genetic abnormalities and molar pregnancies which can lead to such difficult choices to be made once conception has happened.

What is a woman to do when she feels overwhelmed and unable to cope? Many women will simply isolate themselves and not talk about their experiences for fear of being judged by their partner, their family, their friends and acquaintances. Many women come into therapy speaking of how guilty they feel because they should be happy they should be content, they should cope with whatever life is dealing out to them. If they go to their doctor, the fear of many is that they will be placed on some secret list of 'bad' mothers who might have their children removed; or they fear having to take antidepressants, when they don't want to, because they are afraid the tablets may cause birth defects or impact their baby. All of these aspects place women in intolerable dilemmas.

Then we have the difficulty of conventional treatment, using psychopharmacology, which is a controversial subject due to the known and unknown risks of medication in utero and in breast milk and due to adverse effects on the fetus. In those studies where women have been asked about treatment preferences, women prefer psychological therapies rather than pharmacotherapy because it does not involve the risks associated with medication (Fitelson et al., 2011; Kim, O'Reardon & Epperson, 2010). However, in the Western world psychotherapy is not often prescribed. Even though it is possible to place women into therapy groups, which can be just as helpful as one-to-one therapy.

I have included the term distress in this book because it encapsulates the most common forms of mental illness, depression, stress and anxiety. It also captures puerperal psychosis, an unusual but distressful mental health condition at the extreme of mental illness, about which there is little qualitative research. Puerperal psychosis is almost always excluded from research into maternal mental illness as it only affects a very small proportion of postnatal women. However, it is mental illness specifically after childbirth, similar to bipolar disorder. Anxiety and stress are frequently comorbid with depression within the perinatal period, and we know that stress can negatively affect fetal brain development in utero (Schuurmans & Kurrasch, 2013). Many women entering treatment for maternal mental illness speak about their 'distress' and how they are struggling with motherhood and their life in general rather than speaking about being depressed. It is also possible that mothers perceive perinatal illness as a life struggle. Research does not know what causes perinatal depression, stress and/or anxiety as yet and focuses mainly on biomedical explanations. Symptoms are commonly described in nosological terms of classification, with an emphasis on medical diagnostic criteria such as within DSM-5 (APA, 2013), which are not specific to the perinatal period. The actual symptoms may not fit the diagnostic criteria of psychiatric disorders in the DSM. For clarity, it is important that psychotherapists know what the DSM states about maternal mental illness, which is not a lot. It is now included within specific disorders, both of which focus on depressive disorders only, rather than being a disorder in its own right. Whether this is helpful or not is debatable. One could argue either way. What I think is more important for psychotherapists wanting to treat this disorder is to have knowledge about how the medical profession diagnoses it, which they should hold lightly. I think it is helpful to focus on the woman in front of you and how she experiences her illness. Let her tell you what her life and struggle is like, rather than thinking you know what it is like, you don't.

There is also a lack of agreement within the medical profession on the causes of puerperal psychosis, with hormone dysregulation and environmental life stressors being possible factors. However, causal links between puerperal psychosis and hormones, environmental stressors, or even genetics have yet to be identified (Boyce & Barriball, 2010).

DSM V specifiers of perinatal depression – ASA (2013)

Unspecified Bipolar and Related Disorder – 296.80

This category applies to presentations in which symptoms characteristic of a bipolar and related disorder that cause clinically significant distress or impairment in social, occupational or other important areas of functioning predominate but do not meet the full criteria for any of the disorders in the bipolar and related disorders diagnostic class.

With peripartum onset

This specifier can be applied to the current or, if the full criteria are not currently met for a mood episode, most recent episode of mania, hypomania or major depression in bipolar I or bipolar II disorder if the onset of mood symptoms occurs during pregnancy or in the 4 weeks following delivery. Women with peripartum major depressive episodes often have severe anxiety and even panic attacks. Prospective studies have demonstrated that mood and anxiety symptoms during pregnancy, as well as the 'baby blues' increase the risk for a postpartum major depressive episode (DSM-V) (APA, 2013, p. 152).

Unspecified Depressive Disorder – 311

This category applies to presentations in which symptoms characteristic of a depressive disorder that cause clinically significant distress or impairment in social, occupational, or other important areas of functioning predominate but do not meet the full criteria for any of the disorders in the depressive disorders diagnostic class.

With peripartum onset

This specifier can be applied to the current or, if full criteria are not currently met for a major depressive episode, most recent episode of major depression if the onset of mood symptoms occurs during pregnancy or in the 4 weeks following delivery (DSM-V) (APA, 2013, p. 186).

The effects of maternal mental illness

The monetary costs

The first economic study on maternal mental illness, research from the South London Child Development Study, attributed the long-term costs to the mother, the infant, the wider family and the economy (Bauer et al., 2014, 2015). This research focused on perinatal depression and anxiety and showed a substantial cost to the UK economy of around £6.6 billion per annum. This research used decision-analytic modelling, to give the present value of total lifetime costs of perinatal depression and anxiety over the lifetime of mothers and their children. The majority of costs related to the negative effects on the children, with nearly a fifth of those costs borne by the public sector (Bauer et al., 2015). In the USA, the public policy firm Mathematica gave the rate at $14 billion for the year 2017 alone for the cost of untreated mood and anxiety disorders in the perinatal period (Luca et al., 2020). Whilst in Europe, perinatal mental illness is seen to cost around €82,000 per case (McGannan, 2019).

The emotional costs

There are long-term implications of maternal mental illness on the psychological development and mental health of the infant which are gradually being understood but remain inconclusive. Research also exists on the effect on the woman's partner (Leach et al., 2016). Research shows a much greater chance in the likelihood that the infant of a mother suffering from antenatal depression will also develop depression within the infant's lifetime (Lester, Conradt & Marsit, 2013). Negative correlations have been found between perinatal mental illness and the behavioural development of the infant, adverse neurodevelopmental outcomes, low birth weight and pre-term birth, impaired maternal-fetal attachment, trans-generational changes, symptoms of attention deficit hyperactivity disorder and delayed language development in infants of 12 months.

We also know much more about the epigenetic effects on the child of maternal mental illness during pregnancy and in early infancy and childhood 'in some cases, the adult may have absolutely no recollection of the traumatic events, and yet they may suffer the consequences for the rest of their lives' (Carey, 2012, p. 6). Epigenetics is a fast-moving, relatively new field, changing rapidly with breakthroughs in human genome sequencing and DNA methylation. Research in this field suggests a transmission of maternal depression to the fetus through epigenetic mechanisms, which may cause a reprogramming of placental genes, impacting serotonin levels and the hypothalamic–pituitary–adrenal (HPA) axis as well as physiological systems (Lester et al., 2013). This may result in increased cortisol secretion and a reduction in serotonin levels and could make the infant more susceptible to the effects of depression and chronic stress in the postnatal period (Lester et al., 2013). Epigenetic research increasingly shows that antenatal stress affects brain development in utero, which continues into adulthood (Schuurmans & Kurrasch, 2013). Schuurmans and Kurrasch's (2013) comprehensive review showed that maternal distress can negatively impact the unborn fetus' brain, particularly at key neurodevelopmental stages. They concluded that brain development is multi-phasic, beginning in utero and continuing dynamically into adulthood. A negative environment in pregnancy may cause brain development abnormalities which could continue over the lifetime of the person affected. However, they acknowledged that research has yet to uncover how brain disturbances at different time points (prenatal, neonatal, postnatal), combined with the degree of intensity of the disturbance, contribute to the aetiology of conditions and diseases in later life (Schuurmans & Kurrasch, 2013).

As well as the potential effects in utero, the effects on the growing infant post birth are also worthy of consideration due to the mother-infant bond and its necessity to the survival of the infant (Bowlby, 1979; Gerhardt, 2009; Stern, 1985; Winnicott, 1962). Perinatal mental illness can harm the mother-infant interaction in the first year after birth (Gerhardt, 2009). It can also affect a woman physically due to somatisation when a woman has multiple medically unexplained symptoms due to psychological distress (Fink, Rosendal & Toft, 2002). It is now known that chronic and recurrent psychopathology in parents has a detrimental impact on the child, increasing the risk of transgenerational transmission of psychopathology onto the child (Ashman, Dawson & Panagiotides, 2008; Vliegen, Casalin & Luyten, 2014). Epigenetics, neuroscience and biochemistry literature provide a greater understanding of how a disturbed or malfunctioning relationship between mother and infant due to illness either physically or mentally, can affect the infant. It is therefore important that women receive treatment, not only for themselves but also for the sake of the infant. Successful treatment may not only positively affect the future functioning and psychopathology of the child (Cuijpers et al., 2015) but also the mother and wider family.

The prevalence of maternal mental illness

Maternal mental illness occurs within all cultures throughout the world. However, an ongoing tension remains about whether it is a biological or cultural phenomenon. Western cultures tend to attribute it to biological factors, whereas non-Western cultures attribute it to social causes. Feminist perspectives challenge the view that maternal mental illness needs to be medicalised and offer different ideologies and perspectives on its causes. Some believe it is part of a grieving process due to unmet expectations, loss of a sense of self, resentment at the enormous life change and feelings of self-doubt.

Current medical understanding of maternal mental illness is based largely on symptomatology rather than evidence of confirmed diagnoses of maternal mental illness. This may be due to constraints in resources to conduct clinical interviews to confirm diagnoses (Nagandla et al., 2016), or it may be because few medical researchers ask women how they experience their illness, resorting to symptomatology reported by medical practitioners. It is also quite possible that maternal mental illness may be a historic form of mental illness, as many women say they have had some form of mental illness prior to pregnancy. Patton et al. (2015) found historical mental health problems prior to conception in the majority of pregnancies where symptoms of perinatal depression were present. Estimates of relapse in the perinatal period might be as high as 50% of women with a prior diagnosis of severe mental illness (Cohen et al., 2006; Vesga-Lopez et al., 2008). A link also exists between childhood trauma and an increased susceptibility to maternal mental illness within the first six months after childbirth. This resulted in negative child outcomes at 1-year post birth. It is, therefore, possible that women may be more susceptible to mental illness within the perinatal period if they have a history of prior mental illness or trauma. This possible link is important because if women and medical practitioners know this link exists, they are then able to offer timely treatment.

Public Health England (PHE) states that perinatal mental illness affects up to 20% of women from pregnancy to the first-year post birth (Public Health England, 2017). An Australian study using the Depression Anxiety Stress Scale (DASS 21) as well as the Edinburgh Postnatal Depression Scale (EPDS) showed that 29% of women had at least one of the classifications of depression, stress or anxiety, with either an extremely severe, severe, moderate or mild category of mental illness.

World Health Organization (WHO) research on the prevalence of 'common perinatal mental disorders' in low- and middle-income countries found a lack of research evidence in more than 80% of the 112 qualifying countries, 90% of which were the least developed (Fisher et al., 2011). This study highlights both the disparity in quantity of research conducted between countries of differing economic status, and that many countries have no working data. Fisher et al. state that the prevalence in women in low and middle-income countries is substantially higher than the 10% (antenatal) and 13% (postnatal) figures for high-income countries (Fisher et al., 2011), although exact estimates were not given. Their conclusions (corroborated by the WHO Commission on the Social Determinants of Health, 2008) are that prevalence is far greater in women who are the most socially and economically disadvantaged. I have not addressed the prevalence of postpartum psychosis here because it is addressed in Chapter 6.

The evidence reflects only those cases of perinatal mental illness reported within the various health services. As this type of distress can be isolating for women experiencing it and can engender shame, a fear of engagement with services and the sense of being stigmatised, it is probable that the actual levels are well in excess of those reported. Some women may be embarrassed by their illness or indeed fearful that they will be institutionalised or separated from their baby (Boots Family Trust Alliance et al., 2013). Highly distressed women may also have a perceived fear of harming their babies, even though they rarely actually commit abusive behaviours. Mauthner (2002) found that women with postnatal depression become quite passive, isolating themselves from social and intimate relationships, often due to fear and a lack of understanding of their illness. It is also possible that there are many hidden instances of perinatal mental illness that only emerge if there are other issues, for example, child safeguarding issues. Possible barriers to treatment are explored in Chapter 8.

References

APA (2013). *Diagnostic and Statistical Manual of Mental Disorders*, Fifth Edition. Arlington, VA: American Psychiatric Association.

Ashman, S.B., Dawson, G., and Panagiotides, H. (2008). Trajectories of maternal depression over 7 years: Relations with child psychophysiology and behaviour and role of contextual risks. *Developmental Psychopathology*, 20(1), p. 55–77. https://doi.org/10.1017/S0954579408000035

Bauer, A., Parsonage, M., Knapp, M., Iemmi, V., and Adelaja, B. (2014). *Costs of Perinatal Mental Health Problems*. London School of Economics and Political Science, London, UK. Retrieved from https://www.centreformentalhealth.org.uk/publications/costs-perinatal-mental-health-problems [accessed 29.12.21].

Bauer, A., Pawlby, S., Plant, D.T., King, D., Pariante, C.M., and Knapp, M. (2015). Perinatal depression and child development: Exploring the economic consequences from a South London cohort. *Psychological Medicine*, 45, p. 51–61. https://doi.org/10.1017/S0033291714001044

Boots Family Trust Alliance, Netmums, Institute of Health Visiting, Tommy's, The Royal College of Midwives (2013). *Perinatal Mental Health Experiences of Women and Health Professionals*. London: Boots Family Trust.

Bowlby, J. (1979). *The Making and Breaking of Affectional Bonds*. Abingdon: Routledge Classics.

Boyce, P., and Barriball, E. (2010). Puerperal psychosis. *Archives of Women's Mental Health*, 13(1), p. 45–47. https://doi.org/10.1007/s00737-009-0117-y

Carey, N. (2012). *The Epigenetics Revolution: How Modern Biology Is Rewriting Our Understanding of Genetics, Disease and Inheritance*. London: Icon Books.

Cohen, J., Altshuler, L.L., Harlow, B.L., Nonacs, R., Newport, J., Viguera, A.C., Suri, R., Burt, V.K., Hendrick, V., Reminick, A.M., Loughead, A., Vitonis, A.F., and Stowe, Z.N. (2006). Relapse of major depression during pregnancy in women who maintain or discontinue antidepressant treatment. *JAMA*, 295, p. 499–507.

Cuijpers, P., Weitz, E., Karyotaki, E., Garber, J., and Andersson, G. (2015). The effects of psychological treatment of maternal depression on children and parental functioning: A meta-analysis. *European Child & Adolescent Psychiatry*, 24(2), p. 237–245.

Fink, P., Rosendal, M., and Toft, T. (2002). Assessment and treatment of functional disorders in general practice: The extended reattribution and management model – An advanced educational program. *Psychosomatics*, 43, p. 93–131. https://doi.org/10.1176/appi.psy.43.2.93

Fisher, J., Cabral de Mello, M., Rahman, A., Tran, T., Holton, S., and Holmes, W. (2011). Prevalence and determinants of common perinatal mental disorders in women in low- and lower- middle-income countries: A systematic review. *Bulletin of the World Health Organization*, 90(2), p. 77–156. https://doi.org/10.2471/BLT.11.091850

Fitelson, E., Kim, S., Scott Baker, A., and Leight, K. (2011). Treatment of postpartum depression: Clinical, psychological and pharmacological options. *International Journal of Women's Health*, 3, p. 1–14. https://doi.org/10.2147/IJWH.S6938

Gerhardt, S. (2009). *Why Love Matters – How Affection Shapes a Baby's Brain*. Hove: Routledge.

Howard, L.M., and Khalifeh, H. (2020). Perinatal mental health: A review of progress and challenges. *World Psychiatry*, 19(3), p. 313–327. https://doi.org/10.1002/wps.20769

Howard, L.M., Molyneaux, E., Dennis, C.-L., Rochat, T., Stein, A., and Milgrom, J. (2014). Non-psychotic mental disorders in the perinatal period. *Lancet*, November 15, 384(9956), p. 1775–1788. https://doi.10.1016/S0140-6736(14)61276-9

Kim, D.R., O'Reardon, J.P., and Epperson, C.N. (2010). Guidelines for the management of depression during pregnancy. *Current Psychiatry Reports*, 12, p. 279–281. https://doi.org.10.1007/s11920-010-0114-x

Knight, M., Bunch, K., Tuffnell, D., Shakespeare, J., Kotnis, R., Kenyon, S., and Kurinczuk, J.J. (Eds) on behalf of MBRRACE-UK. (2019). *Saving Lives, Improving Mothers' Care – Lessons Learned to Inform Maternity Care from the UK and Ireland Confidential Enquiries into Maternal Deaths and Morbidity 2015–17*. Oxford: National Perinatal Epidemiology Unit, University of Oxford.

Leach, L.S., Poyser, C., Cooklin, A.R., and Giallow, R. (2016). Prevalence and course of anxiety disorders (and symptom levels) in men across the perinatal period: A systematic review. *Journal of Affective Disorders*, 190, p. 675–686. https://doi.org/10.1016/j.jad.2015.09.063

Lester, B., Conradt, E., and Marsit, C.J. (2013). Epigenetic basis for the development of depression in children. *Clinical Obstetrics and Gynecology*, 56(3), p. 556–565. https://doi.org/10.1097/GRF.ob013e318299d2a8

Luca, D.L., Margiotta, C., Staatz, C., Garlow, E., Christensen, A., and Zivin, K. (2020). Financial toll of untreated perinatal mood and anxiety disorders among 2017 births in the United States. *American Journal of Public Health*, 110, p. 888–896. https://doi.org/10.2105/AJPH.2020.305619

Mauthner, N.S. (2002). *The Darkest Days of My Life: Stories of Postpartum Depression*. Cambridge, MA: Harvard University Press.

McGannan, S. (2019). A New PATH to perinatal mental health. In EuroHealthNet Magazine, Behaviour & Addiction, childhood & Adolescence, Edition # 13, Health Inequalities, Mental Health, Policy, Practice. Retrieved from https://eurohealth-net-magazine.eu/a-new-path-to-perinatal-mental-health/

Nagandla, K., Sivalingam, N., Yin, L.K., Abd Majeed, Z., Ismail, M., and Zubaidah, S. (2016). Prevalence and associated risk factors of depression, anxiety and stress in pregnancy. *International Journal of Reproduction Contraception, Obstetrics and Gynecology*, 5(7), p. 2380(9). http://dx.doi.org/10.18203/2320-1770.ijrcog20162132

Patton, G.C., Romaniuk, H., Spry, E., Coffey, C., Olsson, C., Doyle, L.W., Oats, J., Hearps, S., Carlin, J.B., and Brown, S. (2015). Prediction of perinatal depression from adolescence and before conception (VIHCS): 20-year prospective cohort study. *Lancet*, 386, p. 875–883. https://doi.org/10.1016/S0140-6736(15)00018-5

Public Health England. (2017). Better mental health: JSNA toolkit. Retrieved from https://www.gov.uk/government/publications/better-mental-health-jsna-toolkit [13 February 2018].

Schuurmans, C., and Kurrasch, D.M. (2013). Neurodevelopmental consequences of maternal distress: What do we really know? *Clinical Genetics*, 83, p. 108–117. https://doi.org/10.1111/cge.12049. Epub. 6 December 2012.

Stern, D.N. (1985). *The Interpersonal World of the Infant*. New York: Basic Books.

Thurer, S.L. (1994). *The Myths of Motherhood – How Culture Reinvents the Good Mother*. Boston, MA: Houghton Mifflin Company.

Vesga-Lopez, O., Blanco, C., Keyes, K., Olfson, M., Grant, B.F., and Hasin, D.S. (2008). Psychiatric disorders in pregnant and postpartum women in the United States. *Archives of General Psychiatry,* 65(7), p. 805–815. https://doi.org/10.1001/archpsyc.65.7.805

Vliegen, N., Casalin, S., and Luyten, P. (2014). The course of postpartum depression: A review of longitudinal studies. *Harvard Review of Psychiatry,* 22(1), p. 1–22. https://doi.org/10.1097/HRP.0000000000000013

Winnicott, D.W. (1962). The theory of the parent-infant relationship: Further remarks. *International Journal of Psychoanalysis,* 43, p. 238–239.

3 Historical Aspects of Maternal Mental Illness

The history of maternal mental illness is long and dates back to about the 4th century BC and Hippocrates, in his Third Book of Epidemics, where he writes about 'puerperal fever' (a fever lasting more than 24 hours in the first 10 days post birth usually due to infection) (Jones, 1923). Childbirth was, until relatively recently, considered dangerous, with women often dying during labour or shortly after, due to puerperal fever, which was at epidemic proportions in England during the 1760s to 1780s. Giving birth was fraught with fear, pain and difficulty. Pain relief in labour had been possible since the advent of chloroform in the mid-19th century, but anaesthesia during childbirth was not common (Cleghorn, 2021). 'Natural' childbirth with pain was considered physiologically necessary or at least not as painful as women described. These myths about the need for 'pain' or the exaggeration of pain were perpetuated by physicians such as Charles Meigs, an American obstetrician who practiced in the 19th century (Cleghorn, 2021). Meigs was well-known for being completely opposed to any kind of anaesthesia, such as chloroform, in obstetrics, and was even of the belief that it was impossible for doctor's hands to pass on disease, believing that it was an accident that women had puerperal fever and not contagious, as others were suggesting at the time. These myths about lack of pain are even perpetuated today with women often feeling as if they have 'failed' in some way if they receive pain relief, as if this was not normal or natural in giving birth.

Maternal mental illness has remained misunderstood and misdiagnosed for a very long time. Since Hippocrates, there have been many differing interpretations and opinions on the cause of this type of illness. There is still no real agreement, and a split has arisen between more westernised, scientific/medical definitions, which seem paternalistic, and the idea that this type of mental illness is situated in social change, particularly the socio-economic consequences of the modernisation and change in women's roles, a more feminist way of viewing it.

Looking at the history of women's mental illness, and in particular the word 'hysteria' (a term used in the past by doctors to describe emotional excess particularly in females), there is a particular flavour of paternalism running through the diagnosis of maternal mental illness. There has also

DOI: 10.4324/9781003154891-4

been little change in the last centuries about the way in which mothers are depicted. The expectation has been and continues to be that women will be the 'perfect' mother, keeping up with the many household tasks as well as keeping up a fulfilling career. Now, with the increase in the cost of living and the various pressures around the need for material goods, there is also the expectation that she should go back to work as quickly as possible after the baby is born so that she is offering something financially to the family. This is quite a change socio-culturally, as the mother was not necessarily expected to work in the post-war era of the 'idealization of domesticity' (Harrington, 2016, p. 96). This can cause many women to feel caught between social and societal expectations and their own wishes in motherhood, which can be confusing and difficult for women to navigate.

There is also the difficulty around the medicalisation of emotions and the pernicious belief that the mother is to blame for any pathology in the child, which was a post war change brought about by the sense that it was not the state or public policy that was to blame, rather, it was the individual. Mothering has seen a fundamental change from the Victorian times when it was considered normal for a mother to tightly control her children (Harrington, 2016), through to the idea that a mother should be loving and available, responsive and giving to her children at all times, even being the child's 'best friend', which is the idealised vision of parenting more recently. It would appear that since the 19th century, there has been a constant cultural negotiation on what it is to be a 'good enough' mother (Held & Rutherford, 2012) as well as a constant portrayal of the need for the mother to fix herself so that she can get on with being a good mother. This portrayal was also to be seen in the media and the popular press where the baby blues were portrayed as 'normal' and any form of psychiatric illness following childbirth was considered rare. Unsurprisingly, when 'mother's little helper' appeared on the market in the 1960s and 1970s, these tranquilizers became hugely popular as a convenient and efficient way to 'deal' with the difficulties of motherhood (Tone, 2009). These difficulties and their solution even became a subject for mockery by the Rolling Stones in their song 'Mother's Little Helper' in 1966. The tranquilizers then gave way to antidepressants and culturally the baby blues changed and became 'postnatal depression', which was first written about in the USA in the Good Housekeeping Magazine in 1960 (p. 165).

In order to understand the medicalisation of pregnancy and childbirth, it seems important to understand how women's mental health has been portrayed within medicine and society through history, so I will give a very brief description of hysteria.

Hysteria

The history of female hysteria dates back to Ancient Egypt, around 1900 BC, and the Kahun Papyrus (Tasca et al., 2012). For centuries, female hysteria was thought to be due to disorders of the uterus (Cosmacini, 1997; Sigerist, 1951).

In fact, hysteria was considered directly attributable to a malaise of the uterus. This thinking prevailed for centuries, with many advocates such as Aulus Cornelius Celsus (1st century BC) (Penso, 2002), Galen (2nd century AD) (Sigerist, 1951), Trotula de Ruggiero (11th century), possibly the first female doctor in Christian Europe (Tasca et al., 2012), through to Perre Rousell and Jean-Jacques Rousseau, all the way through to Freud. There were those that did not agree, such as René Descartes (16th/17th century), Thomas Willis (17th century) who recognised that hysteria was related to the brain and Thomas Sydenham in 1680 who believed it to have a somatic or psychological explanation, dismissing the theory that it was linked to the uterus (Tasca et al., 2012). From the time of the Ancient Egyptians, the 'cure' for female hysteria was considered to be by fulfilment of inadequate sex life and procreation. Or, advocated by Hippocrates, a pungent smell to return the womb to its natural position, a remedy still seen in Victorian times, when women used smelling salts to recover themselves after an 'attack of the vapours' or rather, heightened emotions. Even Freud continued to believe that hysteria was a female only affliction. The incidence of hysteria in Western cultures declines from the end of Second World War but the incidence of depression and anxiety increases. In 1980, hysterical neurosis was deleted from the DSM-III (Tasca et al., 2012).

With hysteria in particular, it would appear that the only cases reported by doctors and psychiatrists were those experienced by women. Therefore, hysteria was highlighted as a female only condition (McVean, 2017). Yet, research around the end of the First World War clearly shows that men also experienced hysteria in battle (Leff, 1981). Notwithstanding, hysteria still remained in the Diagnostic and Statistical Manual of Mental Disorders, published by the American Psychiatric Association, until 1980.

Insanity and childbirth – Incarceration

Throughout the ages there has been a known link between insanity and childbirth, with even Queen Victoria experiencing a period of low mood after the birth of her second child, documented in December 1841 (Raymond, 1963), which then re-occurred after each of her subsequent seven pregnancies. In France, Dr Jean-Etienne-Dominique Esquirol even set up an asylum for women and wrote his Treatise on Insanity in 1845. This was the beginning of 'puerperal insanity' as a disorder and this type of insanity took hold and flourished (Marland, 2004). Women were incarcerated for reasons of 'Insane by childbirth' or 'Insane by abortion' both in the USA and UK in the 19th century and they had very few rights at that time. Another reason for incarceration was 'suppressed menstruation' and so the female reproductive system became another reason for 'insanity' (Pouba & Tianen, 2006). In a time when *'the correlation between the feminine reproductive system and insanity encouraged a faction of physicians to perform hysterectomies and clitorectomies as a means of restoring mental health'* (Dwyer, 1982), this may be far from surprising. It would appear that the emerging field of psychiatry might have been a useful way of maintaining male dominance.

Puerperal insanity, in particular, was a challenge to the paternalistic view of motherhood; that of domestic bliss and femininity. Women were not the loving, obeying females that men expected, and were seen as a danger to themselves and their children. Puerperal insanity became a term common with medical practitioners as well as in common parlance, with many claiming this to be common and an *'almost anticipated accompaniment of the process of giving birth'* (Marland, 2004, p. 5). Yet childbirth was a woman's most important role and so puerperal insanity needed to be cured. Psychiatry tied together the rigours of reproduction with a woman's weakness and instability, causing a *'meteoric rise and prevalence in the nineteenth century'* (Marland, 2004, p. 6). As psychiatry was almost exclusively a male-dominated profession at that time, this type of insanity became variously interpreted by those with a vested interest in it.

When a woman was incarcerated in an asylum, she was routinely separated from her infant. This practice continued until as late as the end of the first half of the 20th century in the UK. It only stopped when John Bowlby wrote a report for the World Health Organization and highlighted the damage to a child when separated from its mother. His research looked at the impact of maternal deprivation on children who were evacuated in the Second World War. This was the beginning of disagreement about cause and aetiology. The medical, more paternalistic part of the debate being around hormones and medical disorders. The sociological or feminist view being much more around pressures of work, family life and society. The debate on the cause of maternal mental illness continues today.

Postnatal depression and psychosis

The first treatise specifically focused on mental illness in motherhood was written in 1858 by a French psychiatrist, Louis Marcé. This 'Traité de la Folie des femmes enceintes, des nouvelles accouchées et des nourrices' (Treatise on psychoses of pregnant women, and newly delivered and nursing mothers) was not translated into English unbelievably until the 1980s.

After the Second World War, research and treatment of perinatal disorders increased. In 1948 Cassel Hospital, Richmond was the first to admit a mother and her baby with depression that was not considered of psychiatric level. From 1955 onwards, Cassel Hospital then began to admit women and their babies who were experiencing puerperal 'episodes', but not those with psychosis (Humphreys, 2018). There had also been a significant change in knowledge and understanding of the need for a child to be cared for by their mother. John Bowlby's research for the World Health Organization was added to by Winnicott, with his acknowledgement of the way in which a mother could be utterly preoccupied by her baby, calling it primary maternal preoccupation yet normalising it by agreeing that it was natural for a mother to behave in this way with a new baby. Even today, in the 21st century, however, this preoccupation may be seen by some as to be abnormal or even wrong, with women still telling me that there is an expectation for them to give up breastfeeding before they are ready. Many clients tell me also that they are told frequently to 'put your baby down, it will become a rod for your own back'. It would appear that it is difficult to shake off these myths around parenting that come from earlier years.

Around mid-way through the 20th century, there was a distinct change in the way mental illness was diagnosed. Up until the 1950s postnatal mental illness had been seen as a discrete disease entity, with puerperal psychosis believed to be attributed to a toxic-confusional or delirious picture of disease (Coble & Day, 1988). There was also a change in the medicalisation and thinking around mental illness with the advent of psychopharmaceuticals in the 1960s. Mothers needed to regulate themselves by finding a solution to their emotions, rather than learning to adapt to them through time. This solution was medication. The 1960s was also a time of role conflict in motherhood – working versus mothering. In the popular press at this time, mothers were portrayed as disenchanted with being a mother:

> *Half of all new mothers suffered from "disenchantment syndrome" shortly after returning home with the child. They felt an unexpected depression: a sense of being trapped within the house. Here they come into emotional conflict with one of society's "demands": Mothers must always s enjoy their children, and be with them constantly.*

> (Science Digest, 1963, p. 42)

However, finally, a small minority of mothers were being listened to, at least in the UK when for the first time, a community perinatal service was integrated with a small Mother and Baby Unit in the UK in 1974. Dr Margaret Oates opened this two-bed Mother and Baby Inpatient Unit in Nottingham. Dr Oates went on to inspire others to research and treat this type of mental illness and she provided a persuasive argument for more of these types of units to be opened (Humphreys, 2018).

Mother blaming became a part of the 1960s popular discourse, with women castigated for being too involved in their children's lives or else were being pathologised by scientists such as Rene Spitz who seemed to hold the belief that a child's disorder could be traced back to a disorder in the mother (see Spitz, 1965). By the 1970s feminist writing on motherhood was increasing and ambivalence towards motherhood was first beginning to be written (Boston Women's Health Book Collective, 1973). Ann Oakley became the first feminist sociologist to write about postpartum mood disorders in 1980 in two separate books (Oakley, 1980a,b). This was the first time that women were attributing their maternal mood disorders to their disempowerment and the heavy burden of raising children whilst holding down a job or career with little help from their partners. Unsurprisingly, many women began to feel the need to be 'superwoman', juggling their increasing workloads with little in the way of maternity leave and day care, as well as highly unsympathetic employers who still expected them to work long hours.

The Equal Pay Act (1970) and the Sex Discrimination Act 5 years later were supposedly a turning point for Western liberal democracies. Male oppression was being highlighted, mothers were demanding more than simply having children. They wanted to have a worthwhile career too. Women were seemingly advocating their invincibility and their emancipation. However, the career still needed to go on hold or was sabotaged by motherhood. It would appear that in the 1980s women were going to have to choose between their career or motherhood and a feminist backlash began. This led to the highest level of births in the USA ever reported in 1989. However, women were by now an important part in the economies of Western nations, so a move back to the 1950s ideal of the woman in the home did not fit. Instead, the expectation was that they needed to do both. A shift in the framing of maternal illness also occurred with the new belief that postpartum depression was actually caused by physiology (Greenberg & Springen, 2001). This coincided with a move in the UK towards neuroscience and psychology and towards medicalisation of postpartum mental 'illness' with the appropriate medication for everything from postpartum depression to postpartum psychosis and, if necessary, electroconvulsive therapy too. There was also a change in thinking towards attributing hormonal changes as a major cause in postpartum mental illness (Held & Rutherford, 2012). This was not helped by the popularisation and sensationalisation of illnesses such as postpartum psychosis with Martinez, Johnston-Robledo, Ulsh and Chrisler showing that between 1980 and 1998, 32% of articles published about postpartum depression seemed to be written to scare or warn readers about the dangers such as infanticide in such cases (Martinez et al., 2000).

In 1980 the Marcé Society was set up, named in honour of Louis Marcé. This society was originally set up in the UK but has now grown to become a truly international society with members from many different countries. The society is primarily a forum for like-minded multi-disciplinary perinatal specialists to share their research and to disseminate more widely any area of puerperal mental illness, including for fathers, partners and infant research as well as research into treating women experiencing these distressing mental illnesses. Although, in the UK, it was not until June 2014 that the Royal College of Psychiatrists set up a new sub-speciality – Perinatal Psychiatry. Interestingly, this happened after it was decided to remove perinatal mental illness from the categories in the Diagnostic of Statistical Manual of Mental Disorders.

Today there are finally more resources being shared for mothers, and fathers are now finally receiving a small amount of attention, as it is becoming understood that the dads can also experience mental health too, particularly if they are struggling with their own transition to parenthood, or were a witness to a particularly difficult birth and remain traumatised about their experience. There has been a great deal more talk about maternal mental illness due to the pandemic and the huge difficulties women were required to go through, often with no support from loved ones, due to COVID-19 and the difficulties inherent in the medical services with infection control in hospitals. However, science is yet to solve the aetiological mystery of where maternal mental health comes from. Nor is the popular discourse able to fully account for the fact that it is quite possible that women can hold two realities: that they love their children, but equally that they find motherhood really difficult and can feel ambivalence and resentment towards being a mother. None of which makes them a bad mother. I would like to leave the last words to Lisa Held and Alexandra Rutherford from their article 'Can't a mother sing the blues?'

> *Although we began this examination looking for changes in the discourse about postpartum moodiness and mothering over time, we have concluded that certain fundamental ideas remained in place, despite shifts in the scientific, cultural, and political landscapes. [...] The message that motherhood itself should not produce negative emotions, and if it did something was wrong with mother rather than motherhood itself, transcended these shifts [...] Fifty years after the first article on the baby blues, women's complicated experiences of motherhood were still obscured by the overwhelming preoccupation with good mothers as happy others at all cost.* (p. 119)

References

Boston Women's Health Book Collective. (1973). *Our Bodies, Ourselves: A Book by and for Women*. New York: Simon & Schuster.

Cleghorn, E. (2021). *Unwell Women – A Journey through Medicine and Myth in a Man-Made World*. London: Weidenfeld & Nicolson.

Coble, P.A., and Day, N. (1988). The epidemiology of mental and emotional disorders during pregnancy and the postpartum period. In *Psychiatric Consultation in Childbirth Settings*. Boston, MA: Springer. https://doi.org/10.1007/978-1-4684-5439-0_4

Cosmacini, G. (1997). *The Long Art: The History of Medicine from Antiquity to Present*. Rome: Oxford University Press.

Dwyer, E. (1982). The weaker vessel: Legal versus social reality in mental commitments in nineteenth-century New York. In D. Kelly Weisberg (Ed), *Women and the Law: A Social Historical Perspective*. Vol I. Cambridge: Schenkman.

Esquirol, E. (1845). *Mental Maladies. A Treatise on Insanity* (translated by E.K. Hunt). Philadelphia: Lea & Blanchard.

Greenberg, S.H., and Springen, K. (2001). The baby blues and beyond. *Newsweek*, 138, p. 26–29.

Harrington, A. (2016). Mother love and mental illness: An emotional history. *Osiris*, 31(1), p. 94–115. https://doi.org.10.1086/687559

Held, L., and Rutherford, A. (2012). Can't a mother sing the blues? Postpartum depression and the construction of motherhood in late 20th century America, *History of Psychology*, 15(2), p. 107–125. https://doi.10.1037/a0026219

Humphreys, J. (2018). Perinatal psychiatry: Motherhood in mental health services. In G. Rands (Ed), *Women's Voices in Psychiatry: A Collection of Essays*. Oxford, England: Oxford University Press (Chapter 6).

Jones, W.H.S. (1923). *Hippocrates – With English Translation*, Vol 1. London: Heinemann.

Leff, J. (1981). *Psychiatry around the Globe: A Transcultural View*. New York: Marcel Dekker.

Marcé, L.V. (1858). *Traité de la Folie des Femmes Enceintes, de Nouvells, Accounchées et de Nourices*. Paris: Baillière.

Marland, H. (2004). *Dangerous Motherhood – Insanity and Childbirth in Victorian Britain*. Basingstoke, England: Palgrave MacMillan.

Martinez, R., Johnston-Robledo, I., Ulsh, H.M., and Chrisler, J.C. (2000). Singing "the baby blues": A content analysis of popular press articles about postpartum affective disturbances. *Women & Health*, 31, p. 37–56. https://doi.10.1300/JOI3v31n02_02

McVean, A. (2017). *The History of Hysteria*. McGill University, Office for Science and Society. https://www.mcgill.ca/oss/article/history-quackery/history-hysteria

Oakley, A. (1980a). *Becoming a Mother*. Oxford, England: Martin Robertson.

Oakley, A. (1980b). *Women Confined*. Oxford, England: Martin Robertson.

Penso, G. (2002). *Roman Medicine*. Noceto: Essebiemme.

Pouba, K., and Tianen, A. (2006). Lunacy in the 19th century: Women's admission to asylums in United States of America. *Oshkosh Scholar*, 1, p. 95–103.

Raymond, J. (Ed). (1963). *Queen Victoria's Early Letters*, revised edition. p. 74. London: B.T. Batsford.

Science Digest (1963). *Des Moines*, Iowa: Hearst Magazines.

Sigerist, H.E. (1951). *A History of Medicine*. New York: Oxford University Press.

Spitz, R.A. (1965). *The First Year of Life – A Psychoanalytic Study of Normal and Deviant Development of Object Relations*. New York: International Universities Press.

Tasca, C., Rapetti, M., Carta, M.G., and Fadda, B. (2012). Women and hysteria in the history of mental health. *Clinical Practice and Epidemiology in Mental Health: CP & EMH*, 8, p. 110–119. https://doi.org/10.2174/1745017901208010110

Tone, A. (2009). *The Age of Anxiety: A History of America's Turbulent Affair with Tranquilizers*. New York: Basic Books.

4 Pre-Conception, Common Conditions and Confounders

In the process of my work, I have found a few conditions which seem to be most prevalent during pregnancy and within the postnatal period. In no particular order, these are anxiety, stress, distress, depression, postpartum (or puerperal) psychosis and birth trauma. I have chosen to separate birth trauma and psychosis into their own chapters as both are complex areas and warrant having their own voice. I have also added some of the most common confounders later on in this chapter such as addiction, familial factors and the impact of the COVID-19 pandemic.

However, before I begin to talk about these conditions, I would like to go further back to the psychophysiology of the mother created prior to conception, which research is now beginning to show is a time of particular importance. We need to recognise how instrumental this time is, the impact that it can have on the pregnancy, and the ongoing impact on the infant.

Pre-conception and conception

There is now substantial evidence that the mother's prenatal experience will have an impact on the development of her embryo and fetus. However, within health services, little information is offered to women before conception, so most will have no idea about this impact and will not think to or know to change their behaviour accordingly, and indeed may not want to. It is not acceptable for this knowledge to be left unspoken. For some women, it may be of particular importance that they know there is the possibility they can change the environment their fetus will be in during pregnancy.

We know that humans store experience (particularly traumatic experience) at a cellular level (which I will come on to explain). We know that child abuse survivors hold their experience in every aspect of their being (Kirkengen, 2001, 2010). We also know that sexual abuse may be impactful throughout the individual's entire life (Weinstein, 2016). Ann Diamond Weinstein has written at length about the huge amounts of research on pre-conception in her book *Prenatal Development and Parents' Lived Experiences – How Early Events Shape Our Psychophysiology and Relationships*. She writes about the

DOI: 10.4324/9781003154891-5

cellular 'memory' receiving and storing information even before a fetus has a fully functioning brain. This happens through the hormones and substances that pass through the placenta, such as cortisol or endorphins (Verny & Weintraub, 2002). We also know that a female baby is born with all her eggs in situ and that these eggs are impacted by the environment of the mother in utero. So those eggs are already carrying information at a cellular level prior to birth. The placenta also plays a crucial role in the immune system, the neuroendocrine system and the vascular system of both mother and fetus (Weinstein, 2016). This makes sense as it is the placenta that develops in the days post conception, developing its own vascular and cardiovascular system. The placenta transmits everything to the growing fetus:

> *The placenta adapts to the maternal environment and changes both its structure and function with the net result being a change in both substrate supply and to the fetus and the hormonal environment experience by it. The placenta thus assumes an active role in programming the fetal experience in utero which leads to disease in adult life.*
>
> (Myatt, 2006, p. 28)

The placenta may also be implicated in some miscarriages. It is not known fully why some miscarriage occurs. However, the placenta is an area of research due to its fundamental role in pregnancy. Research is being undertaken by members of the Marcé Society and also Tommy's, a charity in the UK, to try and discover the main causes. Many women and couples are left with no knowledge of why they miscarried, which can complicate their grief.

The common conditions

Stress

Stress can have a serious effect on anyone's mental health. Mounting epigenetic evidence increasingly suggests that antenatal stress affects brain development in utero, which continues into adulthood (Schuurmans & Kurrasch, 2013). Some women have suggested to me that they believe their illness begins with the stressors of pregnancy and future concerns about their and their baby's life. The impact of stress on the pregnancy is that it may be a factor in preterm birth:

> *[A] body of research provides evidence that the placenta receives and responds to multiple maternal psychophysiological stress signals, which may result in the activation of labor and birth before full term. ... Neuroendocrine pathways during pregnancy are influential in immune/inflammatory processes that affect fetal development and birth outcomes.*
>
> (Weinstein, 2016, p. 87)

Some of my clients have said their experience of stress was that it grew to a level that became anxiety about many different things. So many women present initially with stress and anxiety that I wonder about the sympto-matic pathway of these two different emotions. It seems that many women initially become caught in a spiral of stress, which causes hyperarousal within their autonomic system, triggering their fight/flight response. This may then enhance their anxiety to a level where they become anxious about other things in their life and begin to feel out of control. This may entail the woman catastrophising about life itself. Also, as a way to counteract stress, anxiety and the uncomfortable feeling of being out of control, some women seem to develop coping mechanisms such as controlling behaviours (Obsessive Compulsive Disorder, or perfectionism, for example), which they use as a way to try to calm their feelings. Others become so overwhelmed that they begin to switch off from life, disconnecting from their partners, family, friends, themselves and their baby.

Freeze/shutdown in pregnancy

As yet, there is an unresearched hypothesis that a mother's freeze shutdown response when pregnant may have an impact on placental and fetal devel-opment due to the reduction in oxygen consumption when this part of the fight/flight autonomic nervous system is activated. There is no definitive confirmation, however, according to Weinstein (2016), we need to take notice that a woman's continued neuroceptive experience of life threat in her environment may impact the placenta and therefore impact the fetus. Clearly, the maternal/fetal/placental relationship is complicated.

Anxiety

Within my practice, this is one of the most common symptoms I see. The anxiety might be anything from concerns prior to the birth, for example, miscarriage or genetic abnormality; health anxieties; fear about the delivery, such as death in childbirth or the baby dying during delivery; and fear about the financial implications of having a baby. Women can be anxious about how to cope with caring for their baby after birth and whether they will live up to their perception of the ideal, perfect mother. Data seems to show that between 13% and 21% of women experience significant anxiety during their pregnancy (Kendig et al., 2017). Some women can tell me why they are anxious, but not all. For example, women with health anxiety, an obsessive sense that they, their baby or their partner will become ill or die at some time in the near future, know that this is what they fear. Others experience death anxiety, the sense that either they will die during the delivery or that their baby will be harmed or will die in the process, is also similarly known. Some have an extreme fear of losing their baby: some are unable to tell me how, and others believe the baby will be snatched or taken away from them by social services. These women will often present as highly functioning, well attached mothers with few apparent difficulties around their infant. Yet, they are consumed with fear, frightened of being judged as not good enough, and fearful of not being able to 'look after' their baby well enough. Some other women I've seen have become convinced their partner will have an affair, becoming almost paranoid with a need to find evidence of culpability. Anxiety can come in many different forms.

What seems to be common throughout all noted anxieties is the fear of impending doom, which can be so strong that the woman feels consumed by it. This fear can have detrimental effects on the woman's relationships with her partner and close family and friends and may also heighten the risk of epigenetic transmission of anxiety, changing the infant's gene presentation which may have negative effects on the infant's own vulnerability to mental illness. Researchers provide many risk factors for anxiety, such as smoking, early delivery, poor social support, poor childbirth experiences, and medical complications in labour. If left untreated, anxiety can affect the infant in many ways, such as having a higher propensity for mental health conditions, impaired cognitive performance, disrupted emotional regulation and impaired attentional processing (Davis et al., 2011; O'Connor et al., 2002a,b).

Not all women are able to speak of their anxiety. Some are unable to voice what they are feeling, other than being 'completely overwhelmed' by what is happening to them. Others sit on the edge of my sofa and literally shake the whole way through their first few sessions as their anxiety is so high. Although these women bodily manifest their distress, they are often unable to offer a narrative about what is distressing them. My sense is that their extreme overwhelm shuts them down, leaving them almost unable to speak and causing them to withdraw into a silent place. These women have little or no ability to regulate their own emotions, experiencing everything as negative and struggling to keep perspective on their life.

Depression

The women I have seen with depression often come because they have been sent by their partner or sometimes by a health practitioner. However, many of them feel so dark and low that coming to therapy can seem too much. When they describe their mood, it is often a description about darkness, using words such as 'hopeless', 'helpless', 'exhausted', 'unable to function, or do anything' and 'completely lethargic'. Symptoms can be impaired thinking, with a mother incapable of finishing her sentences, or unable to find answers to particularly difficult questions, because she cannot think in a way that gives an answer. These mothers don't want to feel this way and often feel guilty that they cannot engage with their baby in the way they feel they should. This lack of engagement can then compound their feelings of depression as they can feel there is no way out, that their baby may be damaged, that they cannot cope, and the enormity of becoming a mother can feel too much.

Often mothers have unrealistic expectations about what they will be able to do once they have given birth. If a woman works in a high achieving career, she may have expectations that she will cope with motherhood easily and keep up the high standards she could achieve prior to birth. Often this is impossible as the demands of a newborn infant, keeping on top of the housework, and the expectation that she should also be enjoying motherhood can seem far from her reality. This can lead to frustration and feelings of being a failure. She also may struggle with the demands of her infant, the feeding, the lack of sleep, the exhaustion and the sense that her role is simply to be a milk bar for her infant. Some women talk about the drudgery of being a mother and how they had not realised it would be this way. Tasks such as nappy changing, feeding herself, making a cup of tea, or even getting up out of bed or off the sofa can feel impossible. Planning meals and going food shopping can seem insurmountable. Some symptoms of depression can seem obvious. However, other signs, such as malnutrition, and self-harm, are not so easy to spot. Women can be in total denial of how unwell they actually are, and this may be because the woman is so determined to show she can cope.

I have often wondered if depression or low mood comes after distress and is a period of shut down that the body/brain goes into after a period of hyperarousal. Certainly, those women who have flat or low mood or who seem numb and find it difficult to speak about their experience seem to me to be in almost a mental shutdown. This does make me wonder if depression may be on a continuum with stress, anxiety and distress and is the body's way of coping with over-arousal. No doubt there will be disagreement by some, after all, I am not a neuroscientist. However, I find it interesting when I talk to women about their experiences that they often talk about high levels of stress and anxiety that lead to depression. Certainly, in my own research, one participant spoke about this 'continuum'. Her symptoms began as stress and anxiety which she talked about as her 'madness of thinking'. She said this tipped into depression and low mood after a period of time (Haynes, 2019), which she attributed to 'mental shutdown'.

The confounders

Addiction

A woman who finds herself addicted to a substance, whatever that may be, may be using the substance to calm herself momentarily. Addiction in pregnancy is a problem due to health consequences for the fetus and newborn infant.

It adds another dimension to treatment as the addiction and the perinatal mental illness both need treating.

The drugs most commonly implicated can be both legal and illegal - alcohol, nicotine, cocaine, amphetamines and opiates, for example. Opiates come in many forms and may be prescribed or bought off the shelf. These types of addictions are a major public health concern, as they not only affect child development but also are a burden on services due to the increasing long-term needs of the infant. In the USA, recent research seems to suggest that just under 10% of the population are illicit drug users (Substance Abuse and Mental Health Services Administration, 2013). Drug use in pregnant women aged 15–44 in America is 5.9% (Substance Abuse and Mental Health Services Administration, 2013), smoking is around 16–17%, and 8.5% of women reported drinking alcohol during their pregnancy (Ross et al., 2015). This highlights that addiction poses a significant problem in maternal mental health.

All drugs (prescribed or illicit) can cross the placenta exposing the fetus, which can cause long-term effects on fetal brain development (Ross et al., 2015). However, drugs also have a direct effect on the placenta and uterus. Dependent upon the substance, this type of addiction can cause low birth weight and premature birth, neonatal abstinence syndrome (NAS) and has developmental and cognitive consequences. Fetal alcohol syndrome (FAS) is caused by alcohol passing through the placenta within the mother's blood and the fetus' inability to process it. It can cause miscarriage and birth defects such a small head size, low birth weight and poor growth, and can also affect the facial features of the fetus. Brain development can be affected causing learning difficulties with maths, memory and speech, for example. The vital organs, hearing and vision can also be adversely affected. Unfortunately, due to the genetic effects (and/or epigenetic), these birth defects are permanent, so a baby with FAS would need to have help through life and is likely to be more susceptible to their own addiction problems and mental illness. The mother's physiology may also be compromised causing a secondary effect such as altered maternal behaviours and increases in the production and secretion of stress hormones. Addiction difficulties for the infant are not confined to the mother, as there are links to paternal addiction and offspring brain development due to epigenetic mechanisms (Goldberg & Gould, 2019).

Single parenting

Many studies show that single mothers experience deleterious conditions due to non-shared care and economic factors caused by the absence of a second income from a partner. Other common confounding factors include lower levels of parental education, poorer socioeconomic status and greater exposure to childhood physical and sexual abuse (Fergusson,

Boden & Horwood, 2007). Divorce can have an impact on the mother due to mental illness and the stress of moving from a two-parent household to a single-parent one. The change in family dynamics can also affect the child, with higher mental health and behavioural difficulties, for example. Co-parenting does offer multifactorial benefits, particularly if both parents play a key role in the children's lives.

Familial factors and lack of support

Familial factors can have a huge impact on pregnancy and child-rearing. These include single-parenting, lack of a familial support network and economic factors such as family hardship and migration, causing a family to live in a culturally and religiously diverse country with very different views of parenting.

In the UK particularly, many more women are bringing up children with little or no family support. There has been a fundamental change in how people live and move around the country due to economic and social factors. People no longer tend to live close to their own families and therefore cannot rely on a family support network to share the burden of childcare. Without the grandparents to help out, the private childcare sector becomes increasingly important. Private childcare is costly, and some women find it more expensive to go back to work than to stay at home and look after their children.

In other cultures, such as Japan and Italy, for example, new parents have negotiated their domestic and working lives by only having one child. In Italy, childcare has become very expensive, and so having more than one child may seem to be prohibitive. For both Italy and Japan, this has meant a decline in population. Culturally, it is still often considered that the burden of domesticity and childcare falls on the woman. School holidays are not easy to negotiate for working women, as the children often get many weeks longer than the woman has for leave. This means a significant gap needs to be bridged for many years. Trying to plug that gap can be difficult, placing economic hardship alongside the stress and strain of bringing up children. Economic hardship often means there is little or no choice but to go back to work and try and find a solution to their childcare needs.

The impact of COVID-19

COVID-19 has led to a fundamental shift in working practices, with many more people working from home. This was due to necessity in the first lockdown and now is from choice. At the time of writing, we are able to go back into our working environments, but there is the ever-present possibility of new COVID variants causing uncertainty.

Perhaps a positive effect of COVID-19 is that fathers are now playing a greater role in their children's lives. It is possible that some men have enjoyed being much more interactive. Some are even choosing to continue to work from home so that their relationship with their children continues. A study by Utrecht University (2020) found that of the fathers they researched, 22% were taking on more care of the children than before (Yerkes et al., 2020). It is quite possible that the evolution of gender roles, which has been changing since around 1965, has been accelerated by the experience of COVID-19 and lockdown. Certainly, more men are asking for help for paternal mental illness than ever before, and there is much more recognition of mental illness within both partners with the advent of children. More forums for fathers have been set up, as well as self-help groups. In countries such as Denmark and Sweden, fathers have been experiencing greater involvement in their children, possibly down to the fact that in Sweden, parents are entitled to 480 days of paid parental leave, regardless of whether a child is born or adopted. Fathers in Sweden tend to take around 30% of all the paid parental leave. However, this does not mean that there is equity in the domestic chores: women still take on the majority of the care for their children (Gnewski, 2019). In Denmark, which also has some of the most generous parental leave, a new proposal (September 2021) sees both parents having 11 weeks of parental leave, as well as an additional 13 weeks that they are allowed to share in the way the parents choose. This is to allow fathers to take a much greater part in the upbringing of their new baby. At present, a Danish father is only able to only take 2 weeks following the birth of his child. In comparison, in a report by UNICEF, the United States has some of the worst maternity leave policies in the world with no national statutory paid maternity, paternity or parental leave (Bryant, 2020).

Conclusion

It is clear that not enough information regarding the importance of psychophysiology prior to conception is available prior to conception. Women need to know their susceptibility to maternal mental illness and the impact of it on their infant and family. Early intervention, even at pre-conception, is preferable. It is also clear that scant information about maternal mental illness exists in the wider domain, making recognition and, therefore, treatment timely. Knowledge is key, as it offers choice. However, this needs to be disseminated to health care providers, as well as to the general public.

A child never chooses to be born, yet it is born with untold potential to act in the world. We need to give every child the chance to honour their potential. This will not happen until humans realise the importance of birth and the meaningfulness and individuality of each and every child.

References

Bryant, M. (2020). Maternity leave: US policy is worst on list of the world's richest countries. *The Guardian*. Retrieved from https://www.theguardian.com/us-news/2020/jan/27/maternity-leave-us-policy-worst-worlds-richest-countries [accessed 29.12.21].

Davis, E.P., Glynn, L.M., Waffam, F., and Sandman, C.A. (2011). Prenatal maternal stress programs infant stress regulation. *Journal of Child Psychology and Psychiatry*, 52, p. 119–129. https://doi.org/10.1111/j.1469-7610.2010.02314.x

Fergusson, D.M., Boden, J.M., and Horwood, J. (2007). Exposure to single parenthood in childhood and later mental health, educational, economic, and criminal behavior outcomes. *Archives of General Psychiatry*, 64(9), p. 1089–1095. https://doi.org/10.1001/archpsyc.64.9.1089

Gnewski, M. (2019). Sweden's parental leave may be generous but it's tying women to the home. *The Guardian*, 10 July 2019. Retrieved from https://www.theguardian.com/commentisfree/2019/jul/10/sweden-parental-leave-corporate-pressure-men-work [accessed 26.10.2021].

Goldberg, L.R., and Gould, T.J. (2019). Multigenerational and transgenerational effects of paternal exposure to drugs of abuse on behavioural and neural function. *European Journal of Neuroscience*, 50(3), p. 2453–2466. https://doi.org/10.111/ejn.14060

Haynes, E. (2019). "Hear Us Speak" – Listening to women's experiences of perinatal distress and the transactional analysis psychotherapy treatment they received. PhD thesis. http://usir.salford.ac.uk/id/eprint/51465/

Kendig, S., Keats, J.P., Hoffman, M.C., Kay, L.B., Miller, E.S., Moore Simas, T.A., Frieder, A., Hackley, B., Indman, P., Raines, C., Semenuk, K., Wisner, K.L., and Lemieux, L.A. (2017). Consensus bundle on maternal mental health: Perinatal depression and anxiety. *Associates in Obstetrics Gynecology*, 129(3), p. 422–430. https://doi.org/10.1097/AOG.0000000000001902

Kirkengen, A.L. (2001). *Inscribed Bodies: Health Impact of Childhood Sexual Abuse.* Dordrecht: Kluwer.

Kirkengen, A.L. (2010). *The Lived Experience of Violation: How Abused Children Become Unhealthy Adults.* Bucharest, Romania: Zeta Books.

Myatt, L. (2006). Placental adaptive responses and fetal programming. *The Journal of Physiology*, 572(1), p. 25–30.

O'Connor, T.G., Heron, J., Glover, V., and the ALSPAC Study Team. (2002a). Antenatal anxiety predicts child behavioural/emotional problems independently of postnatal depression. *Journal of the American Academy of Child and Adolescent Psychiatry*, 41, p. 1470–1477. https://doi.org/10.1097/00004583-200212000-00019

O'Connor, T.G., Heron, J., Golding, J., Beveridge, M., and Glover, V. (2002b) Maternal antenatal anxiety and children's behavioural/emotional problems at 4 years. Report from the Avon longitudinal study of parents and children. *British Journal of Psychiatry*, 180, p. 502–508. https://doi.org/10.1192/bjp.180.6.502

Ross, E.J., Graham, D.L., Money, J.M., and Stanwood, G.D. (2015). Developmental consequences of fetal exposure to drugs: What we know and what we still must learn. *Neuropsychopharmacology*, 40(1), p. 61–87. https://doi.org/10.1038/npp.2014.147

Schuurmans, C., and Kurrasch, D.M. (2013). Neurodevelopmental consequences of maternal distress: What do we really know? *Clinical Genetics*, 83, p. 108–117.

Substance Abuse and Mental Health Services Administration. (2013). *Results from the 2012 National Survey on Drug Use and Health: Summary of National Findings*. Rockville, MD: Administration, S.A.a.M.H.S.

Verny, T.R., Weintraub, P. (2002). *Tomorrow's Baby: The Art and Science of Parenting from Conception through Infancy*. New York: Simon & Schuster.

Weinstein, A.D. (2016). *Prenatal Development and Parents' Lived Experiences – How Early Events Shape Our Psychophysiology and Relationships*. New York: W.W. Norton & Company.

Yerkes, M.A., André, S., Besamusca, J.W., Kruyen, P.M., Remery, C., van der Zwan, R., Beckers, D., and Geurts, S. (2020). 'Intelligent' lockdown, intelligent effects? Results from a survey on gender (in)equality in paid work, the division of childcare and household work, and quality of life among parents in the Netherlands during the Covid-19 lockdown. *PloS one*, 15(11), p. e0242249. https://doi.org/10.1371/journal.pone.0242249

5   Maternal Trauma

Maternal trauma is many different things. It is often attributed to trauma during birth, and of course, this is very much an element. However, I would like to include many other different traumas I see within my work: infertility, tokophobia – extreme fear of childbirth/being pregnant, hyperemesis gravidarum – extreme sickness in pregnancy, miscarriage, termination due to fetal abnormality, stillbirth or neonatal death, rape and sexual abuse, birth trauma and postpartum psychosis.

Maternal trauma is the consequence of any traumatic event from conception through to the postnatal period, as Butler says about trauma, 'this is a past that does not stop being the past, that insists itself on the present, fading and appearing at once' (2006, p. vii). What is vital to understand is that it is the woman's perception that is the most important aspect. Every woman has a distinct perception and a different capacity to cope with trauma. Therefore, it is impossible to equate one woman's trauma to another's, there is no standardised format. Success in treatment is also dependent upon the individual and how they perceive and receive their treatment. In addition, trauma is on a spectrum; two people may experience a similar traumatic event in very different ways. One may show signs of post-traumatic stress disorder (PTSD) and yet another may not experience the event as so traumatic.

One aspect that is important is the way in which the mother may view the infant as part of her trauma. This can be frightening for her, as she may have conflicting views, knowing logically that her baby is not the absolute cause of her feelings, yet also experiencing resentment and a sense that if the baby did not exist, neither would her trauma. Part of the therapeutic contract is to check out these feelings. Some mothers may feel extreme shame around their feelings for their baby and consequently struggle to voice these emotions. Other mothers may be fearful that the baby will be removed from their care if she voices these internal conflicts. Yet another may be scared that she will never love her baby and what the consequences of this may have on her baby's development and social and behavioural skills in later life.

For ease, I am going to split the chapter into specific types of trauma that occur prior to birth, those that may be caused during the birth, and those that occur outside of these particular time frames. Although I have included

DOI: 10.4324/9781003154891-6

postpartum psychosis in the list above, I believe it warrants a chapter of its own (please see Chapter 6).

The first trauma is in pre-conception: infertility. The four main traumas that can occur within pregnancy are tokophobia, hyperemesis gravidarum, miscarriage and termination due to fetal abnormality. I have included this last type of trauma as this is rarely talked about, but parents who go through it are often deeply traumatised by their experience yet feel completely unable to share their grief due to the shame of going through a termination. There are two traumas that occur close to or at birth: stillbirth/neonatal death and birth trauma. Historical rape and sexual abuse can also be re-experienced during birth causing trauma which can be extremely distressful for the woman and the health practitioners who are trying to help her with the birth process. I am always mindful of and listening out for any other elements that can cause trauma, as they can be hidden in the narrative and may be highly individual, yet they are often key to identifying these individual traumatic experiences.

Infertility

Infertility is addressed within Chapter 10 – ethical dilemmas – due to the nature of questions and struggles a couple may have when diagnosed with it. However, in order for completeness, and because this is a form of trauma in pre-conception, I am including it here too.

Between the ages of 20 and 45 years, the estimates for a diagnosis of infertility (failure to conceive within 12 months without contraception – American Society for Reproductive Medicine [ASRM]) is estimated to be between 10% and 15% of women. Infertility is described by the World Health Organization as a global health issue, with statistics showing between 48 million couples and around 186 million individuals struggling with infertility globally (WHO, 2020). There are different factors that cause infertility, and it can occur in men or women. Sometimes, there is no explanation as to why a couple cannot conceive. One element that WHO recognises is the challenge to provide equal and equitable access to fertility care in all countries, particularly for those people living in low- and middle-income countries. Elements that are important are addressing gender inequality – women are often perceived to be the cause of infertility, regardless of them being infertile or not. Infertility can cause stigma, shame, depression, low self-esteem and partner violence. Culturally, in some countries, there can be intense pressure to prove fertility at an early age due to the high value of the ability to bear children. In such areas, raising awareness of infertility, its prevalence and causes can be useful.

Assisted Reproductive Techniques (ART) have been available for around 30 years. However, these are not widely available for all and still remain in the domain of private clinics. There are also laws about the use of ART which are different dependent upon in which country the technique is occurring. This can have implications for those choosing the techniques, which I address more fully within Chapter 10.

Tokophobia

Tokophobia is an extreme fear of childbirth. Interestingly, tokophobia was first written about in 1897 by Knauer and is now becoming more understood within the medical profession and, I hope, within midwifery (Knauer, 1897). There are two types of tokophobia – primary and secondary. The primary type is a morbid fear of childbirth in a woman who has not experienced childbirth before. This can develop as early as childhood or adolescence and may be due to a negative experience, such as watching a television programme or a film, showing childbirth to be a very painful and stressful event. Secondary tokophobia occurs after a traumatic birth experience and can lead to a woman never having another child, no matter what the couple's prior expectations regarding family size might have been. Both types of tokophobia are pathological and are extreme morbid fear. The fear is often so overwhelming that the woman will use several forms of birth control in order to prevent conception. If a pregnancy does occur, some women will feel the need to go through an abortion, as their fear is too overwhelming.

Medically, a woman may be offered anti-depressants as a way to manage her fear. However, it is much more helpful to look at the cause of the fear and to explore it in its entirety. I see women prior to conception who want to fulfil a pregnancy, normally for the sake of their partner who is desperate for a baby. Yet the woman experiences extreme fear even at the thought of being pregnant. When exploring the fear, it may seem to have come out of nowhere. Yet if there is a willingness to explore deeply, there is almost always a cause. This may be a fear of her own death in childbirth or a fear of disfigurement or death of the baby. If there is a plausible reason for the fear, then explore that reason. If it is a fear of death, then explore what it is that makes death seem so possible. Use statistics with caution, as the part of the self who is speaking may be the inner child who cannot understand or make sense of statistics. This inner child does not know how to soothe themselves and is therefore reliant on the therapist to guide them and teach them.

If the tokophobia is so great as to cause the woman extreme distress, it may be worth suggesting she have a conversation with her obstetrician regarding the possibility of having a caesarean section. Fortunately, this is not always necessary. I have had several women with primary tokophobia who have gone on to choose to give birth naturally the second time around. The psychotherapeutic work after the birth of the first child, for these women, was around the sense of 'not doing it right' and their disappointment in themselves. With partner support and also the understanding of a good obstetrician and midwife, these women have gone through their subsequent pregnancies with less anxiety and fear.

Tokophobia may also be for a reason that is at first not conscious to the client. Recently, I worked with Ania who knew she was frightened of becoming pregnant and was unable to contemplate pregnancy due to a pathological fear of needles. She could not think of ever visiting her doctor or going into the hospital for fear of needing to have an injection or blood test. The risk of needles was too high for her. Ania's needle phobia started her tokophobia. She had recently married, however, and her husband wanted her to explore whether she could find a way past her phobia. I used Eye Movement Desensitisation and Reprocessing (EMDR), an extensively researched form of treatment for trauma and PTSD, to see if this would help her phobia which was successful.

Another client, Annette, had a fear of feeling a fetus move in her abdomen. What transpired was that this was around fear of the unknown, and unsurprisingly Annette wanted to remain in control of her environment. Becoming pregnant felt so frightening because she would not be in control of the fetus, as such, and nor would she necessarily be in control of her pregnancy and the ensuing birth. Therapy for this client was about tolerating her fear and letting go of her need to control.

Hyperemesis gravidarum

Between 70% and 80% of all women are sick or feel sick at some stage during pregnancy. For many, this will decrease over time, normally after about 14 weeks. Yet, for some, the sickness continues and can get worse. Hyperemesis is above and beyond the 'normal' experience of sickness as it is extreme nausea and sickness and affects only about 1% of women in pregnancy. It can be dangerous to mother and baby due to dehydration and the woman may need hospitalisation or may become bedbound. It gained attention in the UK due to the experiences of Catherine, Duchess of Cambridge, who was extremely unwell during all three of her pregnancies.

Hyperemesis is a very unpleasant condition and can be extremely debilitating. Many women will feel that their entire pregnancy is spent overwhelmed by being or feeling terribly sick. Some women experience vomiting up to 50 times a day, meaning their whole life is consumed with sickness, leaving them unable to think or do much else. There are differing thoughts about why it occurs, and it would seem that research, as yet, is inconclusive. Medically, it is treated using anti-sickness drugs, replacing fluids, and also administering vitamins B6 and B12.

I include hyperemesis here because I want it to be known about and also because, in my experience, it is helpful for women to talk about what is happening to them. It can be an isolating condition which can cause extremes of emotion, particularly fear that this will continue for the entire 40 weeks of pregnancy. I do not believe it is something that is 'all in the mind'.

Rather, the women I have seen who have experienced this have had specific physiological symptoms. Many have mothers or sisters who also had the condition, and so there may be a genetic link. Also, many have had hyperemesis in their first pregnancy and then come into therapy before their second pregnancy, with fear that the sickness will be there in subsequent pregnancies. There are self-help support groups available, and knowing they are not alone in this condition can be helpful.

Miscarriage

Losing a baby at any stage in pregnancy is an absolutely devastating experience. However, this loss is often discounted by both medical services and within society. This is a type of complex trauma and grief as there is so much hope and fantasy interwoven combined with a sense of utter disbelief when it occurs. Miscarriage is unfortunately a great deal more prevalent than we might think. Most happen in the first 12 weeks of pregnancy, and many are caused by chromosomal abnormalities or by other underlying causes (Tommy's, 2021). Research shows that around 25% of all pregnancies end in miscarriage, and 43% of women who have given birth said they had experienced miscarriage (Cohain, Buxbaum & Mankuta, 2017). This might vary from country to country due to socioeconomic status. The statistics also rise sharply with age. The risk of miscarriage increases to 53% by the age of 45 (Magnus et al., 2019). I have found that women who have experienced miscarriage and come into therapy are common. However, this does not detract from the devastation a woman can feel after experiencing it. It is also important to understand that once a woman has experienced a miscarriage, each subsequent miscarriage increases the risk of another. There also may not be any known cause for the miscarriage which can be distressing and can increase the anxiety felt during a subsequent pregnancy. Research is ongoing into whether miscarriage is caused by a default in the placenta or due to something uncommon, yet specific, such as a 'molar' pregnancy. These arise after the fertilisation of an abnormal egg which implants into the womb lining as a normal zygote would. What occurs then is that the placental cells grow rapidly and begin to overtake the cells of the embryo. This results in a mass of cells which are fluid-filled or rarely can become a cancerous mole (Miscarriage Association, 2020. According to the Miscarriage Association, around one in 600 pregnancies is a molar pregnancy.

The two questions most often asked are 'why did it happen' and 'will it happen again'. In therapy, helping a woman come to terms with not knowing why, nor knowing whether it will indeed happen again can take time. Again, fear is often high and so our work will be around helping the woman try to gain a hold on her fear, exploring it and also exploring what not knowing might mean. Many women can experience a sense of their own failure and will take on total responsibility for the miscarriage. This is not reasonable as there may be many different reasons for the miscarriage.

Working with her around her self-punishment can be fruitful, particularly if she is a perfectionist. Grief can take a long time to dissipate. Couples' work can be both helpful but also a hindrance, dependent upon how the couple function together and the level of ongoing support. Often, each partner is at a different stage to the other, and so this can feel difficult, particularly if one feels stuck in their grief and unable to logically justify it, yet is being asked to do just that. In couples work, one partner may feel angry and upset towards the other, particularly if they feel that the other is diminishing or discounting their grief response. It can feel that they are being asked to move through the cycle of grief more quickly than they feel able to. They might also feel bewildered and confused about how their partner is able to move forwards after the miscarriage. These differences in experience can put a great deal of strain on a relationship and even destroy it. I have worked with couples together initially and then continued to work with the partner who is most affected, helping them to come to terms with their experience. I have also worked with women on their own who did not want their partner to come into therapy, possibly because they would have felt shut down or silenced by their partner. It is really important to listen intently to the woman and not try to move her forward in her process. Having the possibility to explore all the elements that combine to make her fearful and to explore her sense of failure can be really helpful.

Termination due to fetal abnormality

It may cause controversy that I am including this as a type of trauma in pregnancy, which is now known as 'termination for medical reasons' (TFMR). However, in my experience, it is an utterly devastating trauma, which is cloaked often in secrecy and shame. For a woman or couple, it is so hard to be faced with an almost impossible decision about whether to terminate their pregnancy, which may be at a later stage, or to carry the baby to full term, unsure whether the baby may be unlikely to survive the birth experience, or may die very soon after birth. In the UK, around 14 women per day will go through this procedure. DHSC statistics show that 3,183 abortions occurred in 2020 in England and Wales for medical reasons due to 'a substantial risk that if the child were born it would suffer from such physical or mental abnormalities as to be seriously handicapped' (Department of Health & Social Care (DHSC), 2020, p. 10). Another aspect is the guilt these couples can go through and the regret they feel whatever decision they make. It can cause difficulties in future pregnancies through extreme fear about whether this will happen again, and it may cause difficulties in bonding with a subsequent baby. Many couples keep a TFMR completely secret and never tell close family or friends because of their fear that they will be judged about their decision.

Such a form of termination seems to be a taboo subject in parenting. There is also little written about it and very little help for the couple or woman going through it. Yet their loss and grief can be compounded by the reason behind it. Many couples feel silenced by society, as if they are unable to speak about or to grieve their loss or as if they should simply forget about their baby and move on to the next.

Stillbirth and neonatal loss

SANDS: The leading stillbirth and neonatal death charity in the UK.
TOMMY'S: A pregnancy charity in the UK that funds research into
    pregnancy loss.

According to the Office for National Statistics (ONS) in England and Wales, there are around 3.8 births per 1,000 live births that end in stillbirth (after 24 weeks of pregnancy) (ONS, 2021). SANDS, the stillbirth and neonatal death charity in the UK, gives the rate as about 5,000 babies per annum who are stillborn or who die within the first 4 weeks of life (SANDS, 2021). The figure for the US is around 1 in 160 births (24,000 babies) per year (Hoyert & Gregory, 2014). This level has been decreasing in the US recently due to changes in pregnancy care (MacDorman, Kirmeyer & Wilson, 2006). Neonatal loss in the UK (loss in the first 28 days after birth) seems to show a slightly lower rate of 1 in 357 births. Often with stillbirth, there would appear to be no obvious cause with many stillbirths going unexplained. In the US, stillbirth is the loss of a baby at or after 20 weeks of pregnancy. Stillbirth is often classified as early (from 20 to 27 weeks), late (from 28 to 36 weeks, and term (37 weeks onwards). In the UK, there is now a collaboration between Tommy's and SANDS who have together formed a policy unit to gain evidence and advice regarding any changes that could be implemented to reduce the number of infant deaths. They believe that around eight out of ten stillbirths may be preventable with enhanced maternity care (SANDS, 2021).

Stillbirth occurrence appears more frequent with the following factors: ethnicity (black women are more likely to experience stillbirth); age (over 35 years of age increases the likelihood of stillbirth); smoking in pregnancy; multiple births (triplets and quadruplets); in women with a low socioeconomic status; or in women who have had a previous loss in pregnancy (Centers for Disease Control and Prevention, 2021).

Birth trauma

According to research, around 43% of women experience birth as traumatic (Alcorn et al., 2010). It is also clear that trauma is often caused by healthcare providers (now known as 'obstetric violence') and that around 66.7% of women worldwide attribute the healthcare provider as instrumental in the cause of their birth trauma (Reed, Sharman & Inglis, 2017). In her influential book Emma Svanberg cites examples of such violence as '*ignoring mothers*' *knowledge of their own bodies and needs, coercion ("the dead baby card"), and overt violation including examples of women being held down for interventions they did not consent to'* (2019). Trauma during the birth experience can occur in many different ways, either due to a medical emergency or because the experience was unexpected and was perceived as terrifying. PTSD can occur and is often due to an intense fear that either the mother or her baby or both would die during the experience. Symptoms of PTSD are flashbacks, sensate triggers, nightmares, intrusive thoughts and hypervigilance. Some women find it impossible to sleep and this can then exacerbate the situation as extreme lack of sleep can lead to severe mental health conditions, the most severe of all being puerperal psychosis. Women experiencing PTSD will often also experience low mood and an impending sense of doom that something awful might happen again. It can often take a long time for a mother to get over the trauma, and she may get stuck in a cycle of rumination around the birth experience.

Sexual abuse and rape

I have had a number of clients who have struggled with pregnancy after an experience of childhood sexual abuse or rape. In the vignette at the end of this chapter, I describe my work with a client who had been raped in her teens. She had never talked to anyone about the rape. However, it had a profound effect on her ability to engage in any form of sexual relationship, thus impacting the relationships she had.

Treatment for maternal trauma

Dependent upon a woman's experience, I may be treating her for trauma as well as loss and grief. Any kind of grief is difficult, no matter what the circumstances and whether the grief occurs during pregnancy or in the postnatal period. What is important in the therapeutic relationship is to allow the couple to speak and to be truly heard at a deep level. Quite often, the sessions are wrought with significant pain. Offering space and time is important because, for some parents, it can take months for the real depth of despair to be felt in the therapy, and this is often due to the depth of guilt and shame and the belief that it is somehow their fault. Losing this yearned for baby often has the added complication that there may be no apparent reason for the loss of the infant with the couple being told that the miscarriage or fetal anomaly is 'unexplained'. The woman can often feel stuck, particularly in her intimate relationships and also in therapy. Many women talk of this as a sort of madness, and this can be frightening to both the woman and to her family around her.

   Each couple will grieve in their own particular way, with no real pattern to this. A couple who have lost their baby through stillbirth or neonatal loss may have a real desire to cuddle and hold their baby, and this is an important thing for them to do. Some talk about a 'pain' in their arms, which we might think of as the ache of the lack of the baby to cuddle. In couples, there may be a discrepancy in the way they feel their grief, and one may seem to come to terms with the loss quicker than the other. This can cause tension in intimate relationships and may cause friction. It may be that the one who is taking longer to come to terms feels shut down and unable to express their grief for fear of what the other will say.

Neither the maternal instinct nor the hormones go away immediately after loss. This can feel overwhelming for a woman. Some seem to isolate themselves unable to connect with themselves, their partner or the world around them. There can also be such intense feelings of jealousy towards friends or others who are pregnant or who have a healthy newborn. Many women talk about needing to stay completely away from such friends and are often fearful of their intense emotions.

In the same way as for other traumas, EMDR can be helpful for trauma and PTSD symptoms, and if I use EMDR, I always combine it with in-depth psychotherapy. If a woman is experiencing trauma from her birth experience, I believe it is important to explore all areas that 'went wrong', particularly the loss of control a woman may feel because her birth experience did not follow her 'plan'. This can lead to strong feelings of guilt and shame and a sense that she 'did it wrong', particularly if she had set her heart on giving birth naturally, yet an emergency caesarean was needed. There seems to be a strong sense of cultural scripting in many countries that birth is a positive, wonderful and life-enhancing experience. Yet, for many women, this is not the case at all. That sense of the gap between what was expected and what actually happened often needs to be unpicked and explored. Another element that is useful to explore together is the societal myths about 'doing it right' regarding the birth process. Looking at why and how these myths are perpetuated and then helping women to begin to share their experiences of right and wrong in group sessions can be really helpful, particularly if the woman is experiencing a strong level of judgement from her family.

No matter what the cause of the trauma it is important to know how the trauma is being experienced, as this will play a part in how to work with it. There are many elements that may be triggered with trauma including fear, grief, loss of control, intrusive thoughts, catastrophizing, guilt and shame. A focus on helping a mother to bond with her baby when her sense is that the baby is at the heart of her trauma is such an important process.

Clinical vignette

Amy

Amy came into therapy around 12 weeks pregnant with a fear of having her child due to an experience of rape in her early teens. She was married to Cathy and admitted she had at first found any form of sexual relationship really difficult, although she said Cathy had been patient and empathic, which had helped her to come to terms with her experience. Cathy and Amy had chosen to use one of Cathy's eggs, which was fertilised and then placed into Amy, who had wanted to carry the baby. However, now she was pregnant, she was having panic attacks with the thought of giving birth and with fear about her baby moving. This was impacting how she felt about their baby and she was experiencing a level of negative fantasy about the birth and post birth experience.

The work with Amy began with her feelings of disgust at the changes in her body. Unlike many women, who enjoy being pregnant, Amy did not enjoy any part of it at all. As her fetus began to grow, she became more distressed about the lack of control she had over her body and also began talking about her baby almost as if it was something alien. When the baby began to move, she experienced strong feelings of horror and disgust and was desperate for the baby to stop. My experience of Amy was that she had cut off all her feelings from the neck down after her experience of rape, and it appeared she may have been re-experiencing some of the feelings she had felt when she was raped, she often talked as if the baby was 'doing' something to her, almost as if it was purposefully attacking her. Our work became about how to help her tolerate her feelings for the remaining weeks of her pregnancy. We did not focus on the rape at all.

About halfway through her pregnancy, she managed to speak about her deep fear about giving birth, although I could tell that she was fearful about being judged by me. I have seen several women who have re-experienced sexual trauma within the birth process, which is frightening both for the woman and for the medical team around her. I knew it was important for Amy, Cathy and I to explore Amy's feelings and to try and navigate a way through that would be safe for both her and her baby. When it became apparent how deep her feelings went, the complexity of the rape and how it was interwoven with her feelings of disgust, we talked about whether she might ask for a caesarean section for medical purposes. We both thought this was a sensible idea and her obstetrician was happy to listen to her request and subsequently arranged for this to happen. Amy was clearly relieved that she had been listened to, something which began to pave the way for her to speak up more often and be heard, rather than to hide her feelings away and remain silent.

Once her baby was born, our work continued as her feelings of disgust crossed into her experience of breastfeeding. On the one hand, she knew she wanted to breastfeed, yet on the other hand, her repulsion was so intense that she found herself dry retching when she was feeding her son. Again, we explored her options and she attended different breastfeeding sessions to try and resolve her difficulty. In the end, she actually breastfed her son for around six months, which had been a previously unimaginable achievement. She still struggles with her feelings about her body and would prefer for it not to be a part of her. However, as time progresses and our work continues, her feelings of disgust are no longer so intense.

What was really important for Amy at the time of her pregnancy was that we did not explore her rape. We focused on what was happening at the moment in her pregnancy and looked to find ways for her to tolerate her feelings and to find a way through her pregnancy so that her baby could be born safely. She was appreciative of us focusing on the present, as she had high levels of shame around the rape and found it difficult to talk about it. I treated Amy very much the same as I would any client with complex trauma. We did not go into the trauma due to the risk of re-traumatisation and what that might entail for Amy. Instead, we focused on how she was in the moment and how she wanted to be.

References

Alcorn, K.L., O'Donovan, A., Patrick, J.C., Creedy, D., and Devilly, G.J. (2010). A prospective longitudinal study of the prevalence of post-traumatic stress disorder resulting from childbirth events. *Psychological Medicine*, 40, p. 1849–1859. https://doi.org/10.1017/S0033291709992224

Butler, J. (2006). Foreword. In D. Ettinger (Ed), *The Matrixial Borderspace*. p. vii. Nigeria: University of Minnesota Press.

Centers for Disease Control and Prevention. (2021). What is Stillbirth? Retrieved from https://www.cdc.gov/ncbddd/stillbirth/facts.html#ref [accessed 15.11.21].

Cohain, J.C., Buxbaum, R.E., and Mankuta, D. (2017). Spontaneous first trimester miscarriage rates per woman among parous women with 1 or more pregnancies of 24 weeks or more, *BMC Pregnancy and Childbirth*, 17, p. 437. https://doi.org/10.1186/s12884-017-1620-1

Department of Health & Social Care (DHSC). (2020). *Abortion Statistics, England and Wales: 2019 – Summary information from the abortion notification forms returned to the Chief Medical Officers of England and Wales. January to December 2019.* Retrieved from https://assets.publishing.service.gov.uk/government/uploads/system/uploads/attachment_data/file/891405/abortion-statistics-commentary-2019.pdf [accessed 15.11.21].

Hoyert, D.L., and Gregory, E.C.W. (2016). Cause of fetal death: Data from the fetal death report, 2014. *National Vital Statistics Reports*, 65(7), p. 1–25. Hyattsville, MD: National Center for Health Statistics.

Knauer, O. (1897). *Über puerperale Psychosen, für practische Aerzte*. Berlin: Karger.

MacDorman, M.F., Kirmeyer, S.E., and Wilson, E.C. (2006) Fetal and perinatal mortality, United States, 2006. *National Vital Statistics Reports*, 60(8), p. 1–22. Hyattsville, MD: National Center for Health Statistics.

Magnus, M.C., Wilcox, A.J., Morken, N.-H., Weinberg, C.R., and Håberg, S.E. (2019). Role of maternal age and pregnancy history in risk of miscarriage: Prospective register-based study. *British Medical Journal*, 364, p. l869. https://doi.org/10.1136/bmj.l869

Miscarriage Association (2020). Information – molar pregnancy. Retrieved from https://www.miscarriageassociation.org.uk/information/molar-pregnancy/ [accessed 07.06.22].

Office for National Statistics (ONS). (2021). Child and infant mortality in England and Wales: 2019 – Stillbirths, infant and childhood deaths occurring annually in England and Wales, and associated risk factors. Retrieved from https://www.ons.

gov.uk/peoplepopulationandcommunity/birthsdeathsandmarriages/deaths/bulletins/childhoodinfantandperinatalmortalityinenglandandwales/2019 [accessed 15.11.21].

Reed, R., Sharman, R., and Inglis, C. (2017). Women's descriptions of childbirth trauma relating to care provider actions and interactions. *BMC Pregnancy and Childbirth*, 17(21). https://doi.org/10.1186/s12884-016-1197-0

SANDS. (2021). Sands & Tommy's Policy Unit. Retrieved from https://www.ons.gov.uk/peoplepopulationandcommunity/birthsdeathsandmarriages/deaths/bulletins/childhoodinfantandperinatalmortalityinenglandandwales/2019 [accessed 15.11.21].

Svanberg, E. (2019). *Why Birth Trauma Matters*. London: Pinter & Martin.

Tommy's. (2021). Miscarriage statistics. Retrieved from https://www.tommys.org/our-organisation/charity-research/pregnancy-statistics/miscarriage [accessed 21.11.21].

WHO. (2020). Fact Sheets – Infertility. Retrieved from https://www.who.int/news-room/fact-sheets/detail/infertility [accessed 21.12.21].

6   Postpartum Psychosis

Introduction

Postpartum psychosis, defined by the Royal College of Psychiatrists (RCOP) as *'A severe episode of mental illness which begins suddenly in the days or weeks after having a baby. Symptoms vary and can change rapidly. They can include high mood (mania), depression, confusion, hallucinations and delusions. Postpartum psychosis is a psychiatric emergency'* (RCOP, 2018), it is a rare type of psychosis that happens mostly in the first 2 weeks after childbirth. It is also called postnatal psychosis and puerperal psychosis, although all three terms mean the same thing. It is an unusual but frightening and distressful mental health condition at the extreme end of maternal mental illness. It is not common and occurs in about 0.89 to 2.6 per 1,000 women (Vanderkruik et al., 2017) after birth. Different hypotheses exist about why this type of psychosis occurs, although the evidence is inconclusive. There is some evidence to suggest a prior diagnosis of bipolar disorder could be a contributing factor (Boyce & Barriball, 2010). Here, the concern is that the severe changes in mood seen in bipolar disorder may spiral into postpartum psychosis if left untreated. Postpartum psychosis is a serious medical condition and the mother will need help quickly, either through entering an inpatient mother and baby unit to gain the medication and care she needs or through treatment by an outpatient mental health team. Consequences can be extreme such as infanticide and suicide, although this is quite rare, despite media portrayal.

Causation

There is a lack of consensus on the causes, and it has been speculated that environmental life factors, hormones and genetics may play a role. Hormone dysregulation and environmental life stressors are possible factors mentioned in a study by Sharma, Smith and Khan (2004). However, causal links between postpartum psychosis and hormones, environmental stressors, or even genetics (Jones & Craddock, 2001) have yet to be identified (Boyce & Barriball, 2010). There seem to be two elements of causation which are 1) predisposition or susceptibility; 2) a 'trigger'. The RCOP gives a useful table

DOI: 10.4324/9781003154891-7

of information quantifying the risk of postpartum psychosis based on personal and familial history. Examples of personal risk factors include, in particular, bipolar disorder (especially Type 1) and other schizoaffective disorders. The familial factors include a mother/sister with a history of postpartum psychosis (RCOP, 2018). Hormones, environmental factors/stressors and lack of sleep could interact with a genetic predisposition. Lack of sleep seems to be a significant feature of the illness and may be involved in causation as well as being a symptom. In academic research into maternal mental illness, postpartum psychosis is almost always excluded as it only affects a very small proportion of postnatal women and is considered extreme mental illness.

The symptoms of psychosis are different to low mood and depression and are sometimes described as mania. There are different types of symptoms:

- hearing voices
- hallucinations – seeing things that are not there
- delusions about things that are actually not true
- pressure of thoughts and speech, such as talking extremely fast, which may seem chaotic and non-sensical to others listening
- Withdrawal and isolation – with some women seeming unable to speak
- loss of appetite which may have been due to extreme low mood
- real difficulties with sleep and sometimes not sleeping at all for days at a time
- confusion and behaviours that are totally out of character
- Extreme euphoria – expressing exuberance that everything in the world is fantastic and wonderful
- Or the other extreme – narrating that they believe they are dead and are not in the world anymore

My first experience of a mother believing she was dead was when working in an MBU (Mother and Baby Unit) with a woman who was utterly convinced she and her baby had died in childbirth and were, in fact, in hell. This experience has never left me, as it was the first time I had seen postpartum psychosis. This woman had a profound impact on me and was the reason I chose to specialise in this area. I realised how traumatised she was once the psychosis began to subside. At the time, there was no psychological therapy offered in the unit to help her with her trauma nor outside once she had left the unit.

Women with postpartum psychosis do not necessarily know how unwell they are. For example, a mother came one day with extreme euphoria who felt the whole world was fantastic. Yet being with her, I sensed that something was really not quite right. It felt like she was in a fantasy world, chattering volubly. This woman had no insight into her illness at all. In fact, she told me how wonderful it was not to sleep for days, as she could achieve so much more. It is often close family and friends that spot the warning signs that something is not quite right. A lack of insight is often associated with psychosis and other different disorders such as personality disorder, substance addictions, or depression, for example (Reddy, 2016). It is important to highlight next of kin and family and their role in providing a history of symptoms in order to establish a diagnosis. They are also likely to be involved with the ongoing care and support for the woman, especially if she is not admitted into the hospital. However, it should be emphasised that the family may also need support to help them cope with looking after the mother and her infant through this distressing time.

This type of psychosis can be extremely frightening for the woman and her family. It can cause trauma and it may take a long time to come to terms with. Some women are terrified it will return if they choose to have another baby. They may choose to remain with just one child, the fear of risking another episode being too great to cope with. However, it is treatable, and it does not necessarily mean that the woman will have postpartum psychosis again, although about 50% of women do, with the birth of a subsequent baby (Di Florio et al., 2013; Jones et al., 2014; Wesseloo, Kamperman & Munk-Olsen, 2016). What may be helpful to know is that women with a diagnosis of bipolar disorder and other mental health disorders are at greater risk of experiencing this type of psychosis (Wesseloo et al., 2016).

I have included a small amount of research into women's lived experiences of postpartum psychosis as they are so often excluded in any type of research project.

Experiences of postpartum psychosis

Forde, Peters and Wittkowski (2020) conducted a metasynthesis of qualitative research on women's experiences of postpartum psychosis and the factors women believed were involved in their recovery. They found 15 studies which captured the views of 103 women and found 4 main themes and 13 subthemes. The four main themes were:

1 Experiencing the unspeakable (which encompassed 'trapped in an insane mind', fear and hopelessness, how the illness came 'out of the blue', and the impact on caring for and bonding with the baby
2 Loss and disruption (which encompassed the challenge to the woman's sense of self, guilt from missing out, and powerlessness)
3 Realigning old self and new self (which encompassed how this was a non-linear process, how the woman made sense of and integrated her experience and the 'return to normal life'
4 Social context (the impact on family relationships, with healthcare professionals and societal expectations to 'snap out of it')

They highlight how unique the experience of this type of psychosis is and that the pathway to recovery is not linear. They recommend an individualised approach to treatment which would include long-term psychological and psychosocial support, with further staff training and service development also needed. Of the 15 studies they found, I have highlighted 5 below.

Engqvist et al. (2011) explored the experience of postpartum psychosis using women's narratives gained from specific internet sites offering information, support and assistance to women suffering from postnatal mental illness. The purpose of their study was to enhance the quality of care and to decrease the suffering of women with psychosis. The narratives explored were those freely accessible on those specific sites. They found four main themes:

1　Unfulfilled dreams (which encompassed disappointment with the delivery, pervasive guilt and paranoia, and inability to care for their infant)
2　Being enveloped by darkness (overwhelming fear, being in an 'unreal' world, being 'controlled' by someone or something, and confusion/disorganised thinking)
3　Disabling symptoms (sleeplessness, being unable to concentrate, feeling 'ill at ease', and self-destructive behaviour)
4　Feeling abandoned (from infant, paranoia and distrust of everyone, detachment from the world and from their infant, dissatisfaction with care)

In a small-scale study, Engqvist and Nilsson (2013) explored the accounts of seven women about their first few days of psychosis. The authors discovered five main themes:

1　Being in an unreal world
2　Loss of sleep
3　Infanticidal ideation
4　The transition from wanting their baby to not wanting their baby
5　Suicidal ideation

For women experiencing it, postpartum psychosis was seen as a time of darkness and despair. Lack of sleep, particularly in the first days after giving birth, was considered of great significance as the first sign of psychosis, which is corroborated by Sharma et al. (2004). The study, although small, was useful in highlighting the importance of intimate support through partner or close family and their role in early detection and recovery support.

In another small-scale study, Glover (2014) interviewed seven women who had been diagnosed with psychosis. Their research discovered four main themes:

1　The route to psychosis
2　The experience of unspeakable thoughts and an unacceptable self
3　A need to 'snap out of it'
4　The women's perception of the causes of their psychosis.

They discovered that women attributed their psychosis to physiological changes in pregnancy and childbirth, yet the narrative of their experiences often began prior to conception, with them citing life difficulties, distress and anxieties as part of their journey into psychosis. The study concurs with other studies (Doucet, Letourneau & Blackmore, 2012; Robertson & Lyons, 2003) that psychosis is a biomedical event. However, they also believe there is a need to continue to seek a more holistic, multi-dimensional explanation of psychosis rather than to constrict it solely to the biomedical dimension.

Robertson and Lyons (2003) analysed women's experiences of psychosis and discovered three main themes:

1 women separating their psychosis from other mental health disorders, believing that it was different
2 An over-riding sense of loss during this time and post-psychosis
3 How women had to negotiate their social roles and changes to their relationships with others during this time, and the difficulties these caused.

The research highlighted the stigma and isolation women felt when going through psychosis, as well as the subsequent pathology placed upon their emotions once the psychosis was over, which continued the stigmatisation. It highlighted the sense of anger and isolation these women felt suffering from such a rare condition. This caused women to direct their anger towards health professionals due to the perceived lack of information and support for themselves and their families. More recently, Engqvist et al. (2011) reported similar findings that women may still be experiencing a sense of abandonment when they go through psychosis.

Heron et al. (2012) interviewed five women on discharge from an in-patient mother and baby unit to address the risk of maternal suicide on discharge. They sought to understand the difficulties the women faced and their experiences of the illness and to build a picture of support needs. Full recovery from psychosis was viewed as a long and difficult process. The emotional reactions women felt from an episode of psychosis were similar to those found by Robertson and Lyons (2003), particularly in relation to loss. Consistent with the research from Robertson and Lyons (2003), Heron et al. found the women reported a lack of knowledge, information and support from health professionals and again this was equated with 'lack of power'. This research, although of a small sample size, was in-depth and rich with detail from the women's experiences.

All the studies highlight how women perceived their psychosis, where they believed it originated, how disabling their experiences were, their sense of the 'unspeakable thoughts' they experienced and how this led to them feeling unacceptable, and how isolated and abandoned they felt within their illness. The gap in knowledge both from a biomedical perspective on what causes this illness and the minimal knowledge of women's experiences would benefit from much broader, deeper studies.

Psychotherapy and postpartum psychosis

I wish to be clear that I am not advocating psychotherapy as a suitable treatment for a woman who is actually experiencing a psychotic episode. There are psychotherapists who are also psychiatrists who do work with schizophrenia and psychosis, such as the TA psychotherapist and psychiatrist Zefiro Mellacqua, who has written eloquently about his work in his book *Transactional Analysis of Schizophrenia: The Naked Self.* However, I am not a psychiatrist and I would be stepping out of my own capability as a professional to work this way. If someone is having a psychotic episode, this is a medical emergency and they need to be seen by a psychiatric team specialising in treatment. However, this does not mean that I would not be able to be with and 'hold' a woman experiencing this. My experience of women who were having a psychotic episodes was during my placement, working in an inpatient mother and baby unit. The role I had was one of being present with the woman, listening to her and offering reassurance rather than giving therapy. It is doubtful whether a woman would be giving informed consent to psychotherapy when she was experiencing psychosis, so it would not be ethical. I have also had one client who came to me when they were experiencing psychosis and two who contacted me by phone at the beginning of their psychotic episode. Due to risk to their safety, I contacted their doctor for them on their behalf, with them present in the room or via telephone. Each was then seen by their local Crisis Team (Crisis Resolution and Home Treatment Team). This possibility of contact with the doctor is part of my initial contract with clients. At the point of contacting their doctor, I am clear to ask the client again for permission. We normally do this in discussion, and with psychosis, I am still careful to discuss this with the client. I prefer the client to be in the room with me when I am speaking to their doctor so that they can clearly hear what I am saying. All three women were showing high levels of fear and extreme levels of hyper-arousal. What is interesting is that all three either had familial conflicts occurring, as well as extreme sleep deprivation, at the time of their psychosis, or they had extreme paranoia about their infant being removed by their partner or a family member. When reading Mellacqua's work, he talks about Paul Federn's observation: 'Every psychosis is consciously or unconsciously focused on conflicts or frustrations in family life' (Federn, 1952, p. 120). My experience of working with psychosis is limited in comparison to Mellacqua's. However, with those I have treated for the trauma after their psychosis, I would say that family conflicts or frustrations around the birth have been present at a lesser or greater degree in each one.

I have seen a number of women for psychotherapy after discharge from an inpatient mother and baby unit, and I would describe each one as severely traumatised from their experience. Most found the severity of their illness impacted their ability to bond and connect with their baby, which was part of their distress, as was their sense of isolation in their illness, and disconnection from themselves, their partners, their babies, their families and the wider world.

I have also had clients with a history of bipolar disorder who went on to have a psychotic episode during our long-term work together. For those women, my role has been one of remaining as a constant background presence through their experiences. Mostly, these women have been admitted voluntarily for a short-term stay into a mother and baby inpatient psychiatric unit. Each time I have remained available to them if they wanted to speak to me for any reason, and on their return home, our work has continued. Each of these women has spoken of my knowledge of them before their episode began and as a 'witnessing other' during their experience and afterwards, which seemed to be helpful and reassuring to them. They will often ask me how they were before and whether they have changed. Sometimes I am asked about their stay in hospital, and many have little recollection of their time in hospital.

All these women are often traumatised by their experiences. They feel marginalised and often mortified by what has happened to them. Coming to terms with their experience takes time and can take years. Often, they describe being attacked by their illness. They talk about the psychosis as if it is separate from them and I have had a sense of them splitting the psychosis away as if they can keep themselves safe from its malevolent force.

In particular, working with someone who has medical experience and also has had psychosis can be difficult. There is an acute shame, which comes from knowledge of the condition, the medication prescribed, and fear of stigmatisation from work colleagues. One doctor I worked with said she was absolutely devastated about her psychosis and struggled for many years to come to terms with what had happened.

One particular difficulty is the medication prescribed often means a woman needs to stop breastfeeding immediately due to the possibility of harm to the infant as the medication may be transmitted into breastmilk. This can add to the woman's sense of being 'not good enough', or for some, a sense of utter failure as a mother. For some women who really want to breastfeed, having to stop can feel disastrous and seems to compound their trauma. They talk about having lost connection with their baby, which they feel as a huge loss. Others can feel anger at having to give up something they were passionate about doing.

Many women are totally confused by their behaviour during the psychosis and are frightened by themselves, as they are unable to understand why they might behave in such uncharacteristic ways:

> *I was, it was like a different person, but I knew I was doing it but I couldn't control it, (pause) erm doing all different random things, thinking that I'd been followed.*
>
> 'Jane' (Haynes, 2019)

There is also a sense of an alteration of time, with some clients telling me they lost track of time in hospital and were unable to tell me how long their psychosis had lasted.

> *It felt like a lost time, there was one day actually that I saw the clock and it actually went to different times.*

'Jane' (Haynes, 2019)

Some women do experience a sense that they are dying, or they have died. Jane (above) felt that she was going to die and related being totally convinced that she would die imminently.

I believe that psychotherapy is a suitable treatment for the aftermath of postpartum psychosis, in the period when the woman, and her infant, have been discharged from inpatient care yet is still struggling to come to terms with what happened to her. Often these women have been prescribed high levels of medication such as antipsychotics. Medication can also make the woman feel lethargic, not herself, and one of my clients talked about her husband describing her as 'the lights are on, but nobody's home' due to his sense of her being 'vacant' on the medication. The medication can cause women to put on a great deal of weight. This is not helpful when they are already feeling a sense of low esteem and, for some, abject misery.

Amongst other relational techniques of psychotherapy, I have found using creativity useful when working with the trauma of postpartum psychosis. Please see Chapter 14 for a more detailed description and a client vignette, where I use a creative object within our psychotherapeutic frame as a way of helping the client to realise she was shifting and changing, which lessened her fear that another psychotic episode was looming and inescapable.

References

Boyce, P., and Barriball, E. (2010). Puerperal psychosis. *Archives of Women's Mental Health*, 13(1), p. 45–47. https://doi.org/10.1007/s00737-009-0117-y

Di Florio, A., Forty, L., Gordon-Smith, K., Heron, J., Jones, L., Craddock, N., and Jones, I. (2013). Perinatal episodes across the mood disorder spectrum. *JAMA Psychiatry*, 70, p. 168–175. https://doi.org/10.1001/jamapsychiatry.2013.279

Doucet, S., Letourneau, N., and Blackmore, E.R. (2012). Support needs of mothers who experience postpartum psychosis and their partners. *Journal of Obstetric, Gynecologic and Neonatal Nursing*, 41, p. 236–245. https://doi.org/10.1111/j.1552-6909.2011.01329.x

Engqvist, I., Ferszt, G., Ahlin, A., and Nilsson, K. (2011). Women's experience of postpartum psychotic episodes – Analyses of narratives from the internet. *Archives of Psychiatric Nursing*, 25(5), p. 376–387. https://doi.org/10.1016/j.apnu.2010.12.003

Engqvist, I., and Nilsson, K. (2013). Experiences of the first days of postpartum psychosis: An interview study with women and next of kin in Sweden. *Issues Mental Health Nursing*, 34(2), p. 82–89. https://doi.10.3109/01612840.2012.723301. PMID: 23369119.

Federn, P. (1952). *Ego Psychology and the Psychoses*. New York: Basic Books.

Forde, R., Peters, S., and Wittkowski, A. (2020). Recovery from postpartum psychosis: A systematic review and metasynthesis of women's and families' experiences. *Archives of Women's Mental Health*, 23(5), p. 597–612. https://doi.org/10.1007/s00737-020-01025-z

Glover, V. (2014). Maternal depression, anxiety and stress during pregnancy and child outcome; what needs to be done. *Best Practice & Research Clinical Obstetrics and Gynaecology*, 28, p. 25–35. https://doi.org/10.1016/j.bpobgyn.2013.08.017

Haynes, E. (2019). *"Hear Us Speak" – Listening to women's experiences of perinatal distress and the transactional analysis psychotherapy treatment they received*. PhD thesis. http://usir.salford.ac.uk/id/eprint/51465/

Heron, J., Gilbert, N., Dolman, C., Shah, S., Beare, I., and Dearden, S., et al. (2012). Information and support needs during recovery from postpartum psychosis. *Archives of Women's Mental Health*, 15, p. 155–165. https://doi.org/10.1007/s00737-012-0267-1

Jones, I., Chandra, P.S., Dazzan, P., and Howard, L.M. (2014). Bipolar disorder, affective psychosis, and schizophrenia in pregnancy and the postpartum period. *Lancet*, Nov 15, 384(9956), p. 1789–1799. https://doi.org/10.1016/S0140-6736(14)61278-2

Jones, I., and Craddock, N. (2001). Familiality of the puerperal trigger in bipolar disorder: Results of a family study. *American Journal of Psychiatry*, 158, p. 913–917. https://doi.org/10.1176/appi.ajp.158.6.913

RCOP (2018). Help and Information – Puerperal Psychosis Retrieved from https://www.rcpsych.ac.uk/mental-health/problems-disorders/postpartum-psychosis?searchTerms=postpartum%20psychosis [accessed 21.12.21].

Reddy, M.S. (2016). Lack of insight in psychiatric illness: A critical appraisal. *Indian Journal of Psychological Medicine*, 38(3), p. 169–171. https://doi.org/10.4103/0253-7176.183080

Robertson, E., and Lyons, A. (2003). Living with puerperal psychosis: A qualitative analysis. *Psychology and Psychotherapy – Theory Research and Practice*, 76, p. 411–431. https://doi.org/10.1348/147608303770584755

Sharma, V., Smith, A., and Khan, M. (2004). The relationship between duration of labour, time of delivery, and puerperal psychosis. *Journal of Affective Disorder*, 83, p. 215–220. https://doi.org/10.1016/j.jad.2004.04.014

VanderKruik, R., Barreix, M., Chou, D., Allen, T., Say, L., Cohen, L.S., Barbour, K., Cecatti, J.G., Cottler, S., Fawole, O., Firoz, T., Gadama, L., Ghérissi, A., Gyte, G., Hindin, M., Jayathilaka, A., Kalamar, A., Kone, Y., Lange, I., Magee, L.A., Mathur, A., Binns, A.M., Morgan, M., Munjanja, S., Gichuhi, G.N., Petzold, M., Sullivan, E., Taulo, F., Tunçalp, Ö., von Dadelszen, P., on behalf of the Maternal Morbidity Working Group. (2017). The global prevalence of postpartum psychosis: A systematic review. *BMC Psychiatry*, 17(1), p. 272. https://doi.org/10.1186/s12888-017-1427-7

Wesseloo, R., Kamperman, A.M., and Munk-Olsen, T. et al. (2016). Risk of postpartum relapse in bipolar disorder and postpartum psychosis: A systematic review and meta-analysis. *American Journal of Psychiatry*, 173, p. 117–127.

7 Narratives of Maternal Mental Illness

One of the things I find most striking in my work and learning about this type of illness is how specific it is to each woman. This specificity is the way a woman perceives her illness, and it is not necessarily the same as her symptomatology. Externally, women may appear to have the same symptoms, yet each woman defines her illness in her own particular way. Nor are the narratives the same, although they do have similarities. This puts me in mind of a quote by the philosopher Hannah Arendt regarding our uniqueness, which fundamentally captures how I feel about each of the women I see: '*Nobody is ever the same as anyone else who ever lived, lives, or will live*' (1958, p178). I have tried to capture some of the different descriptions to give a flavour of them, much of which is evidence-based. When there is research, I have referenced it too, so that it is clear which is research, and which is my thinking. It is this specificity of illness that I think is crucial to address in treatment and may be why more formulaic styles of treatment with a prescribed protocol may not offer a positive long-term prognosis.

Even though there is this specificity, I also see clear repeating themes. These themes overlap and contribute to each other. For example, a woman who tells me she is a 'failure at breastfeeding' may also perceive herself as a 'failed mother', which precipitates feelings of guilt and shame, and can lead women to isolate from family and healthcare professionals. It is important to draw attention to the insufficient research into women's lived experience of maternal mental illness. What research there is most often focuses on the postnatal period and on depression only. The chapter ends with a brief clinical vignette called 'the fatherless mother'.

Lack of knowledge

Lack of knowledge is a theme I hear frequently. I split it into two distinct parts: the woman's, and the healthcare professional's lack of knowledge. Women specifically tell me they have a gap in their knowledge about perinatal mental health conditions. Many have heard of postnatal depression, but know little or nothing about anxiety, postpartum psychosis or obsessive behaviours, for example. When coming for therapy, one of the aspects that most clients want,

DOI: 10.4324/9781003154891-8

and need is a greater knowledge about what is happening to them. Knowledge reduces fear and also offers validation and reassurance that they are not 'imagining it' or 'going mad'. This theme of lack of knowledge in women is backed up by research from Raymond et al. (2014), Tobin, Di Napoli and Beck (2018), and Ugarriza (2002). Women tell me that they would like more knowledge about pregnancy, childbirth, and raising their child, yet many say this is difficult to find from authors they would trust. I think this lack of knowledge highlights how women often remain silent about birth and mental illness experiences, particularly if they are negative. This may be for fear of 'putting off' a friend or colleague who is pregnant and upbeat about her news. It may be due to shame which is difficult to share because it does not resemble societal expectations of what she 'should' be experiencing. Or it may be a sense that 'everyone' experiences negative emotions, and they are normal. This lack of knowledge is perpetuated through the ongoing myths of motherhood, the sense that we should be 'natural' mothers, and are adapted for childbirth and breastfeeding, and that we should instinctively know how to do it. This is a cultural, sentimentalized and incorrect myth perpetuated at length, which is harmful. It also is the myth which helps to keep women silent.

More surprisingly, I often hear an underlying thread of a lack in the knowledge of health professionals, particularly those at the front end of perinatal care. This is backed up extensively by research (Furber et al., 2009; Highet et al., 2014; Wittkowski et al., 2017). Women who have sought out help from their doctor or health visitor talk about the health professional not having concrete knowledge of the full breadth and depth of this illness. Many health professionals continuously refer to it only as postnatal depression, even though women may not be exhibiting symptoms of depression at all.

There is a general lack of awareness and insufficient recognition of anxiety disorders in the perinatal period. This lack of knowledge leads to confusion among women with anxiety or trauma, as their symptoms don't fit the information they have been given, causing a sense of alienation. It also shows a lack of understanding in the medical profession that this illness is much more than simply depression. Highet et al. (2014) felt this lack of understanding of the complexities of illness was in part due to the higher profile of postnatal depression. Some health practitioners will not often see the sharper end of illness, such as postpartum psychosis, for example, so may not understand it and be scared of its consequences.

Additionally, women talk about their frustration in the lack of time, care and understanding they have been shown. As a result, women struggle to open up to their health care professionals and do not trust them enough to divulge their illness fully, as evidenced by the research by Coates, Ayers & de Visser (2014) and Tobin et al. (2018). This is understandable. When a woman is struggling with feeling unwell yet is offered only short appointment (often now by telephone), within which to try to describe exactly how she is feeling, it is unsurprising that she will often give up, rather than persevere. It can seem too hard to try and be understood. This is backed up by Dr Helen Stokes-Lampard, the president of the Royal College of General Practitioners, who in 2017 said that GP consultations in the UK were too short for people with complex health needs (Duncan & Levett, 2017).

Exhaustion

Exhaustion is a theme that comes up a great deal, with mothers telling me they feel utterly exhausted. Unfortunately, they often report that health practitioners simply normalise lack of sleep. Yes, new parents do not sleep well. However, lack of sleep is on a spectrum. Some people function OK on very little, whereas others can become seriously unwell quite quickly with little sleep, often compounded by struggling with eating or drinking enough, or taking care of their own basic needs.

To be clear, lack of sleep plays a role in maternal mental illness. We know that sleep deprivation is a form of torture. Yet, some medical professionals seem to believe it does not warrant attention and are reluctant to prescribe medication. This is understandable on the one hand – if a mother is breastfeeding, she might not want to take a benzodiazepine, for example. However, when a mother is unable to function due to severe emotional exhaustion, the choice may be only between a short-term prescription for sleep medication or severe mental illness. And sometimes, it can be that stark a choice, particularly when a mother is on the edge of mania due to significant lack of sleep. Even one or two nights of decent sleep can make a huge difference to a woman's ability to cope.

We should also consider iron deficiency within exhaustion. I have seen several women who have been diagnosed with an iron deficiency during pregnancy and also postnatally, or who have had relatively severe bleeding at birth, yet who have received little in the way of treatment. This leaves them feeling utterly exhausted for extended periods of time. Iron deficiency in pregnancy can increase the risk of lack of fetal growth and early labour (VanderMeulen, Strauss, & Lin, 2020) and postnatal haemorrhage (American Society of Anesthesiologists (ASA) Press Release, 2019). It can make the woman feel utterly drained, with little capacity to enjoy pregnancy or motherhood. For some iron-deficient women, even the simplest parts of childcare can seem almost impossible. This is not of benefit to the woman, nor her infant and family, and may be the beginning of withdrawal and isolation as a protective mechanism. There are different types of iron deficiency, so if a woman is complaining of severe exhaustion in therapy, it is important to suggest she gets her iron levels measured through a simple blood test and receives suitable treatment.

Loss in the transition to motherhood

One element I regularly hear about is women's sense of loss and frustration in their transition to motherhood. There are numerous changes in pregnancy and post-birth, so it is unsurprising that some women experience this as a loss of some part of themselves, as reported both by Highet et al. (2014) and Nicolson (1999). This loss and frustration can reinforce their dissatisfaction in pregnancy and motherhood, as there has often been a fantasy that they will continue as they were pre-pregnancy (for example, energy, libido, body shape and identity). Nicolson highlighted identity, work, time, relationships, the loss of their own body and friendships as factors in the sense of loss and grief a woman can feel. Writing in 1999, she talked only about postpartum depression, and her argument was that it was not a pathological condition, even though the longstanding myths of motherhood continued to frame it this way.

Loss of identity is a huge factor in maternal mental illness, particularly with a first child. The women I see often hold onto their idealisation of motherhood when they are first pregnant, determined that their pregnancy and their experience will be straightforward, with a simple birth plan, no medication and a 'natural', easy labour. Some do have it easy. However, this idealisation is a set up to fail, because pregnancy, birth and motherhood are often not easy. Women in general are also impeding new mothers, by remaining silent about their experiences. Forewarned is often forearmed. In the 21st century, it is high time we spoke about the difficulties that can occur and help women to become more proactive in gaining knowledge they say they lack. Health care professionals could make it easier for women to share their experiences as a part of information dissemination. Women could then ask questions, and question the answers they receive, particularly if those answers are from those who purport to 'know'.

The gap between fantasy and reality – Unmet expectations

When reading much of the research into women's narrative experiences, I found a wide gap between the expectations and the reality of motherhood. I would argue that this gap is fuelled by the cultural myths of motherhood that continue to perpetuate even today in the 21st century. These myths play a huge role in reinforcing the sense of failure and frustration women feel once they have given birth. Yet the myths are often spurious, as Shari Thurer writes about in her book *The Myths of Motherhood*. These feelings of failure and frustration lead to guilt and shame and a real sense of stigmatisation.

When coming to therapy, many women seem to have a perceived need to grieve the loss of their particular fantasy of motherhood. I would add that women who have gone through artificial reproductive techniques (ART) may feel the gap between fantasy and reality even more sharply, particularly if the process of becoming pregnant has been long and difficult. This gap results in unmet expectations. Often women cling on to a fantasy of the mother they thought they would be, which is shattered by the reality of who they experience themselves as being. This disparity between fantasy and reality can lead to huge disappointment and may also knock a woman's confidence in her ability to mother. It can leave women feeling overwhelmed due to their continuous struggle and the lack of time they have to achieve everything they think they should. Research by Beck (2002), Choi et al. (2005), Mollard (2014) and Read, Crockett and Mason (2012) highlights this disparity between reality and fantasy.

Many women talk in therapy about their unmet expectations of motherhood. Breastfeeding and giving birth naturally are the most cited expectations I hear. Women often feel an intense pressure to breastfeed, from family, healthcare professionals and also from society (Coates et al., 2014; Gao et al., 2010; Haga et al., 2012). There is also the continued mantra of 'breast is best', particularly in healthcare settings. Although breastfeeding has a huge amount of evidence of its benefits for the newborn infant, this presupposes that all women can breastfeed, which is not true. My question would be, best for whom? It is naïve to think that just because a woman has breasts that she will produce milk of sufficient quantity, and be able to latch her baby on suitably, so that both feel OK. This mantra makes women who cannot breastfeed feel high levels of guilt and anxiety as they are unable to give their baby 'the best start in life'. This can compound feelings of failure, as they are not able to be 'the perfect goddess mother'. Also, some women find the idea of breastfeeding abhorrent and are phobic. These women feel pressured to feed but have a repulsion towards it, which may have been due to rape or sexual abuse in childhood. I find it more helpful to open a dialogue up about what the difficulties or misgivings are, and what is best for both mother **and** baby. Focusing only on the baby's needs excludes the mother and can make her feel like her only role is as a womb and a milk bar.

The pressure to give birth 'naturally' is another expectation that many women have and then struggle with, if this does not happen. Most women seem to use the term 'natural childbirth' to mean giving birth without medication. Those women who then undergo an emergency C-section or who have epidurals tell me that they have not done it 'right', triggering feelings of loss and disappointment.

There is quite a bit of research about this perceived inability to meet the high expectations of being the 'perfect mother' or 'good mother' (Beck, 2002; Chan et al., 2009; Gao et al., 2010; Haga et al., 2012; Mauthner, 1999; Mollard, 2014; Staneva, Bogossian & Wittkowski, 2015; Stone & Kokanovic, 2016).

Attacked

I find it really interesting how often women narrate their experience of mental illness as if they are being 'attacked' by it, as if it is some malevolent external force. I find this particularly with clients who have experienced postpartum psychosis. When we speak about this sense of this external force, I often gain a sense that, for the woman, this illness came 'out of nowhere'. As if suddenly they were ill, when prior to this they were not. The plea I hear time and time again, including in my own clients and research, is the need to go to a time 'back then', prior to the pregnancy, when there was nothing wrong with them. In my own research, this theme was also present in some of the participants. My clients talk cognitively and logically that they know that this was in fact an internal process, yet at a deep psychological level, they still narrate this attacking force as external to them.

It does have a kind of feeling that it was something out of me, but obviously it wasn't. But it has that kind of (pause) it's so foreign.

('Sarah' in Haynes, 2019, p. 206)

Even a woman who experienced this illness many years before still seemed unsure of what it was that had happened to her and was still searching for answers and reassurance from me. Some women even describe their illness as 'attaching itself' to them. This seems to describe an inability to control it, which is often the factor they found most scary.

Disconnection

Many women talk of feeling a sense of disconnection from themselves, their babies and the outer world, particularly when their mental illness is at its height. This disconnection can also feel like being abandoned in their illness, with a sense of extreme loneliness and isolation. This is apparent in many parts of their lives, from intimate relationships, familial relationships, relationships with their baby, medical relationships and relationships with friends and the wider world. This sense of abandonment is also described by Stone and Kokanovic (2016). When a woman comes into therapy, and seeks help, she is seeking connection through a relational act, that of speaking about her illness.

Disconnection and the sense of being overwhelmed manifest through silence within this illness, with women unable to, or choosing not to, voice their difficulties. Silence is one of the biggest problems as it is one of the most significant barriers to treatment (see Chapter 8). Some women literally choose not to talk to anyone for years, although family and friends may have a sense that something is very wrong. I have had clients tell me they have never spoken about their illness, until they came to therapy. This can be years later. In fact, the longest a woman remained silent until she finally spoke to me was 40 years. It is not uncommon for me to see women 5, 10 or even 20 years after their illness. They often come to see me about something else, a daughter going through a difficult pregnancy, perhaps, and when we track back, they talk about what happened to them when they were giving birth to their daughter. This transgenerational aspect is common and needs to be explored within the therapeutic process. It can also be really useful to explore the woman's own birth story, and that of her mother and grandmother, if she knows them. This can help with unlocking her own story of birth, and also highlights the transgenerational aspect, whereby women going through severe maternal mental illness may have had a mother/grandmother who also experienced it.

Within recent research, many women talk about how lonely or isolated they felt with perinatal mental illness (Abrams & Curran, 2009; Bennett et al., 2007; Raymond et al., 2014; Stone & Kokanovic, 2016; Tobin et al., 2018). This is possibly because they felt they needed to hide their illness. In their meta-synthesis of nine studies, Knudson-Martin and Silverstein (2009) found it was isolation, and the inability to talk about or express themselves emotionally, that maintained and supported their postnatal depression. A meta-synthesis by Staneva et al. (2015) highlighted the strong sense of disconnection and dissociation women felt with themselves and their babies. In my own work, I find that disconnection comes hand in hand with low mood and depression. It is not that the woman wants to disconnect, it is more that she displays symptoms of disconnection after experiencing extremes of distress.

Health anxiety

I use the term 'health anxiety' to describe the behavioural manifestation of a type of mental illness I see quite frequently in women. This is normally a fixation on her own or her infant's health, which spirals upwards as her illness progresses. If this is not addressed, it can transfer into increasing levels of anxiety and may culminate in panic attacks or even psychosis. Some women may have a conviction they are about to die, and this may feel extremely real for them, even if the medical profession reassures them that there is nothing wrong. Health anxiety can also be a fear of dying during the birth process (mother and/or baby). These feelings and convictions can be extremely powerful. When women talk about their health anxiety, they seem to know at one level that their fear is irrational, yet they are often absolutely convinced about it. It may be difficult for family and friends to hear, particularly if the anxieties are perceived as illogical.

Some women may not express health anxiety in such a heightened way yet may talk about how they feel they 'cannot go on'. This may or may not be suicidal ideation, so it always needs to be investigated thoroughly. It might be more of an expression that the body and mind cannot cope with the level of anxiety they are experiencing at the time. It can be useful to ask whether they cannot go on, or whether they want the situation to stop. As yet, there does not appear to be any research literature that acknowledges or explores health anxiety as a symptom of perinatal mental illness. However, such research would be invaluable.

Madness

My clients often talk about feeling a kind of 'madness' when describing some of their symptoms. This might be a sense of madness in their thoughts (the 'madness of thinking'), intrusive thoughts which they find particularly distressing or a sense that their madness is bizarre. When we explore this together, some women can acknowledge how distorted and abnormal their behaviour or thinking is, yet they are unable to control these thoughts. This can lead to them questioning their ability to mother, their fear of harming the baby or being harmed themselves or they might worry unnecessarily about the baby. Such feelings of 'madness' or being 'psychotic' are supported in research by Stone and Kokanovic (2016), Beck (2002), Bennett et al. (2007) and Tobin, Di Napoli and Beck (2018). When women experience intrusive thoughts, these can become intolerable, and as a way of trying to cope, may lead to compulsive behaviour.

Seeking help only at crisis level

Many women can find it extremely difficult to seek help and may only finally ask for help when they have reached crisis level. Often this will be because they are petrified they will be abandoned by their loved ones and ultimately that their children will be taken away. This fear can be so intense that it can keep a woman silent for years. Fear of losing a child due to maternal mental illness is supported in a huge amount of research (Bilszta et al., 2010; Boots Family Trust Alliance et al., 2013; Byatt et al., 2013; Edwards & Timmons, 2005; Jarrett, 2016; Knudson-Martin & Silverstein, 2009; Mollard, 2014; Nakku et al., 2016; O'Mahen et al., 2015; Staneva et al., 2015; Stone & Kokanovic, 2016; Tobin et al., 2018). Unfortunately, women are still fearful of losing their child, because they are unable to read the research, or do not know it exists and therefore do not know that this removal of a child rarely happens. Other aspects might be cultural, such as an inability to disclose feelings, or difficulty in admitting their illness to family and friends due to fear of engendering cultural stigma and shame.

Even clients I see who have medical knowledge – doctors, midwives, health visitors – find it difficult to speak out even though they have professional knowledge of perinatal mental illness and possibly psychosis. These women tell me they fear being shamed and stigmatised at work and talk about how their illness might not be perceived well, which I find extraordinary. These women work within the medical profession, yet the one place they speak about that they believe they will not find the understanding and compassion they need is precisely in the system they work in. This only serves in prolonging their silence, and a need to externally project a façade of being OK, when they are anything but OK.

My hope is that this is now beginning to change. However, it is long overdue. In the UK, there has been a glacially slow change in focus towards mental illness within the NHS. It is possible that the COVID-19 pandemic has finally highlighted just how rife mental illness actually is. Whether this helps the medical professionals I see, I am unsure. It is a different matter treating people for mental illness, than treating internal staff members. Any change in attitude would be a relief, and definitely not before time.

Masks

Women often relate to me a need to wear a 'mask', or to hide behind one, not able to show how they really feel. This is very much a need to hide all the stigma and shame, embarrassment and guilt they feel, pretending to be someone else and hiding behind a false persona. For some, they want to show a 'brave face' to the world and continue as if all is well. This behaviour is particularly found in women who are immigrants or have refugee status (Schmied et al., 2017). They hide their illness due to the fear of their status, and of their baby being removed from them, instead 'putting on a happy face' as a way of keeping their level of denial and delusion going. Women feel intense guilt and shame around feeling unwell and many women will go to great lengths to try and hide their feelings, outwardly appearing OK, yet inwardly feeling increasing distress. This does not help them at all, as it can lead to a paradox – they tell me they hide their illness, yet also tell me that their family and friends do not understand the severity of their illness or are not around when needed. Even when women spend time with their immediate family, they will speak of their inability to acknowledge and voice their distress with those around them. Quite often, the family colludes in this, possibly with a hope that if it is unspoken, then it will eventually pass. This is a naïve position to take, as women can go for years with this form of mental illness. Some women will also have their own internal messages of not being able to ask for help, or are in total denial, acting to everyone as if nothing is wrong, even though they may be experiencing psychosis.

The consequence of all these different themes is silence, stories unspoken, difficulties unseen and struggles unaided. Hearing about all these different themes is important, but it is also useful to hold them lightly, not to try and put the woman into a box and make assumptions about what she is feeling and experiencing. There are almost undoubtedly many more themes that I could generate. However, I am not sure it is helpful to swamp the reader with vast quantities of narrative. What I would say is not to make assumptions, to think you know what the mother is feeling. Those assumptions will almost certainly be off the mark. Nor is it helpful to make any fast decisions about how the treatment should be planned and how it will progress. Each treatment plan will follow its own path, one that is discovered and formed together.

I have chosen the case example below in order to show how the cause of maternal mental illness may be due to a specific incident in a woman's life, which could have occurred many years before. With each client, it is important to seek out their own specific cause, whatever that might be. Sometimes the client will know. More often, they will not know the cause and it will become apparent part way through the journey together, as it did with this client, Rachel.

Client vignette

The fatherless mother – Rachel

Rachel came because she was experiencing huge anxiety about putting her baby, Sophia, down. She said she had an easy pregnancy. It was from the point of giving birth, her anxiety levels went through the roof. When I asked what her fear was, she said that something terrible would happen to Sophia, that she would be taken away from her, somehow. She found it almost impossible to go to sleep without Sophia beside her, and continuously checked that Sophia was still alive. She told me she would often wake convinced that Sophia was dead, having dreamed just that. Another symptom was intrusive thoughts of harm befalling her baby. Each time she walked down the stairs with Sophia in her arms, for example, she would have immediate intrusive thoughts that she would trip and fall, crushing Sophia and killing her. If she put Sophia in the car, she would have thoughts that they would be involved in a catastrophic car accident.

We discovered the cause of her catastrophising was tied up with the loss of her father. Rachel lost her father suddenly, in the middle of the night when she was twelve. She woke up one morning, and her parents were nowhere in the house. She said she remembered how quiet the house was, and described it as almost eerily quiet, with just herself and her younger brothers. She said she knew something had happened, but she did not know what. Later she discovered her father had suffered a heart attack in the middle of the night and her mother had gone with him to the hospital. He then died in hospital from another more severe heart attack a few hours later. When Rachel told me about the loss of her father, she showed no sign of distress or grief and narrated her story to me in a flat, calm way, as if this was a perfectly normal thing to happen during her teenage years. The only clue I had was my countertransference, which was a sense of agitation and weight in my chest, when she told me her story.

A breakthrough in our work came when Rachel began to learn how she cut off her feelings as a way to protect herself. I noticed that there was a great deal of incongruence between how she spoke about her story and what she was narrating. Rachel had learnt to negate her feelings from her mother, describing her as a strong figure, who had little time for emotions, particularly sadness, and after his death, Rachel said her father was rarely mentioned again.

There was another turning point when Rachel began to realise that it may have been around the time of her father's death that her anxiety began, and she remembered not wanting to leave her mum, fear of going to school, struggling to sleep due to experiencing night terrors, dreaming she had woken up to find that her whole family were missing, and no matter how hard she looked for them, she could not find them. The more we began to explore being a teenager, the more Rachel began to realise the impact of her father's sudden death. Each fear she had seemed inextricably linked to catastrophic death, sudden, out of the blue and unforeseen.

I was surprised that Rachel was not concerned about her husband's safety. I had wondered about this absence in her fear. Rachel joked about choosing her husband because he was safe. He was a police officer. We talked about how their relationship was very much gendered. She portrayed him as the protector, and her as the stay-at-home mother, which she was happy to be. Unlike some other mums I had seen, she did not want to go back to work at all and told me she was happy to be at home with her daughter. I wondered with her if this was because home meant a semblance of safety and control for her. It seemed to me that Rachel was trying desperately to reproduce a fantasy of how her childhood should have been. Almost as if this would somehow change the past.

Although she did not talk about it at first, about part-way through our work together, Rachel admitted she had a tendency to be obsessive and had a need to control, telling herself that if she could control all aspects of her life, then bad things would not happen. This was an unconscious game she played with herself, over and over again, completely unaware. She was quite shocked to learn she did this. To counteract her need to control, I brought in as much spontaneity and creativity as possible into our sessions and encouraged her to bring spontaneity into her life with her daughter and husband. She found playing with Sophia very difficult, particularly imaginative play and admitted to having no idea what play really was about. One of the things she struggled with most was mess. Painting, playdoh, any kind of toy that was messy was a problem for her as she could not bear to have toys and puzzles on the floor. Our work shifted to helping her let go of this need for absolute control, to learn how to find joy in playing with Sophia, rather than simply tidying up after her.

Our work drew to an end when Rachel realised her anxiety had reduced substantially. In fact, she said she no longer felt anything like the 'dark cloud of doom' and admitted she could not remember when she had last catastrophised. She was also able to voice what she was experiencing, as well as to ask for help, and for what she needed, at the moment. She noticed how her need for control had released its iron grip, and how her connection with Sophia was strong. In our last session, she reflected on how she had been when Sophia was born and recognised her behaviour as engulfing. She still had moments of terror that something had happened to Sophia, yet she was able to manage those moments better, calming and soothing herself, something she had never been able to do before. One of the last things she told me was that she realised she did not need to be anxious anymore, acknowledging to herself and to me that she was internally generating this anxiety. Our work lasted for two years.

I worked with Rachel in the same way as I do with all my clients, beginning with reducing her distress to enable her to think more clearly, moving onto our therapeutic alliance and attachment, then exploring and interpreting her experience (see Chapter 13 for an in-depth description of treatment). My work is compassionate, but it is much more than this. A client needs more than compassion alone to be able to change. They need to be able to explore their shadow side, those unconscious dynamics that drive whatever it is they are feeling. We need to be able to go there with our clients, to uncover the terrifying unknown with them. In this regard, Bill Cornell highlights this by saying 'Awareness of unconscious experience necessitates an encounter with otherness, differentness. The essence of interpretation, the impact of an interpretation, is precisely in the fact that what is observed and spoken by the other is not within the client's experience of himself or herself' (2013, p. 282).

References

Abrams, L.S., and Curran, L. (2009). "And you're telling me not to stress?" A grounded theory study of postpartum depression symptoms among low-income mothers. *Psychology of Women Quarterly*, 33(3), p. 351–362. https://doi.org/10.1177/036168430903300309

American Society of Anesthesiologists (ASA) Press Release. (21.10.2019). Women with anemia twice as likely to need transfusion after caesarean delivery. Retrieved from https://www.asahq.org/about-asa/newsroom/news-releases/2019/10/8-anemia-after-cesarean [accessed 29.11.21].

Arendt, H. (1958). *The Human Condition*. Chicago: University of Chicago Press.

Beck, C.T. (2002). Postpartum depression: A metasynthesis. *Qualitative Health Research*, 12, p. 469–488. https://doi.org/10.1177/1049732021299120016

Bennett, H., Boon, H., Romans, S., and Grootendorst, P. (2007). Becoming the best mom that I can: women's experiences of managing depression during pregnancy – A qualitative study. *BMC Women's Health*, 7, 13. https://doi.org/10.1186/1472-6874-7-13

Bilszta, J., Ericksen, J., Buist, A., and Milgrom, J. (2010). Women's experiences of postnatal depression – Beliefs and attitudes as barriers to care. *Australian Journal of Advanced Nursing*, 27(3), p. 44–54.

Boots Family Trust Alliance, Netmums, Institute of Health Visiting, Tommy's, The Royal College of Midwives. (2013). *Perinatal Mental Health Experiences of Women and Health Professionals*. London: Boots Family Trust.

Byatt, N., Biebel, K., Friedman, L., Debordes-Jackson, G., Ziedonis, D., and Pbert, L. (2013). Patients' views on depression care in obstetric settings: How do they compare to the views of perinatal health care professionals? *General Hospital Psychiatry*, 35(6), 598–604. https://doi.org/10.1016/j.genhosppsych.2013.07.011

Chan, S.W., Williamson, V., and McCutcheon, H. (2009). A comparative study of the experiences of a group of Hong Kong Chinese women and Australian women diagnosed with postnatal depression. *Perspectives in Psychiatric Care*, 45(2), p. 108–118. https://doi.org/10.1111/j.1744-6163.2009.00211.x

Choi, P., Henshaw, C., Baker, S., and Tree, J. (2005). Supermum, superwife, supereverything: Performing femininity in the transition to motherhood. *Journal of Reproductive and Infant Psychology*, 23(2), p. 167–180. https://doi.org/10.1080/02646830500129487

Coates, R., Ayers, S., and de Visser, R. (2014). Women's experiences of postnatal distress: A qualitative study. *BMC Pregnancy & Childbirth*, 14, p. 359. https://doi.org/10.1186/1471-2393-14-359

Cornell, W.F. (2013). Relational group process – A discussion of Richard Erskine's model of group psychotherapy from the perspective of Eric Berne's theories of group treatment. *Transactional Analysis Journal*, 43(4), p. 276–283. https://doi.org/10.1177/0362153713515180

Duncan, P., and Levett, C. (2017). How long do you get with your GP? Doctors' consultations times – in data. *The Guardian*, 10.02.2017. Retrieved from https://www.theguardian.com/society/datablog/2017/feb/10/how-long-do-you-get-with-your-gp-doctors-consultation-times-in-data [accessed 22.12.21].

Edwards, E., and Timmons, S. (2005). A qualitative study of stigma among women suffering postnatal illness. *Journal of Mental Health*, 14(5), 471–481. https://doi.org/10.1080/09638230500271097

Furber, C.M., Garrod, D., Maloney, E., Lovell, K., and McGowan, L. (2009). A qualitative study of mild to moderate psychological distress during pregnancy. *International Journal of Nursing Studies*, 46, p. 669–677. https://doi.org/10.1016/j.ijnurstu.2008.12.003

Gao, L.-L., Wai-Chi Chan, S., Liming, Y., and Xiaomao, L. (2010). Experiences of post-partum depression among first-time mothers in mainland China. *Journal of Advanced Nursing*, 66(2), p. 303–312. https://doi.org/10.1111/j.1365-2648.2009.05159.x

Haga, S.M., Ulleberg, P., Slinning, K., Kraft, P., Steen, T.B., and Staff, A. (2012). A longitudinal study of postpartum depressive symptoms: Multilevel growth curve analyses of emotion regulation strategies, breastfeeding self-efficacy, and social support. *Archive of Women's Mental Health*, 15, p. 175–184. https://doi.10.1007/s00737-012-0274-2

Haynes, E.F. (2019). 'Hear Us Speak': Listening to women's experiences of perinatal distress and the Transactional Analysis psychotherapy treatment they received, PhD thesis, University of Salford, http://usir.salford.ac.uk/id/eprint/51465/

Highet, N., Stevenson, A.L., Purtell, C., and Coo, S. (2014). Qualitative insights into women's personal experiences of perinatal depression and anxiety. *Women and Birth*, 27, p. 179–184. https://doi.org/10.1016/j.wombi.2014.05.003

Jarrett, P.M. (2016). Pregnant women's experiences of depression care. *The Journal of Mental Health Training, Education & Practice*, 11(1), p. 33–47. https://doi.org/10.1108/JMHTEP-05-2015-0023

Knudson-Martin, C., and Silverstein, R. (2009). Suffering in silence: A qualitative meta-data-analysis of postpartum depression. *Journal of Marital and Family Therapy*, 35(2), p. 145–158. https://doi.org/10.1111/j.1752-0606.2009.00112.x

Mauthner, N. (1999). Feeling low and feeling really bad about feeling low: Women's experiences of motherhood and postpartum depression. *Canadian Psychology*, 40, p. 143–161. https://doi.org/10.1037/h0086833

Mollard, E.K. (2014). A qualitative meta-synthesis and theory of postpartum depression. *Issues in Mental Health Nursing*, 35(9), p. 656–663. https://doi.org/10.3109/01612840.2014.893044

Nakku, J.E.M., Okello, E.S., Honikman, D.K.S., Ssebunnya, J., Ndyanabangi, S., Hanlon, C., and Kigozi, F. (2016). Perinatal mental health care in a rural African district, Uganda: A qualitative study of barriers, facilitators and needs. *BMC Health Services Research*, 16, p. 295. https://doi.org/10.1186/s12913-016-1547-7

Nicolson, P. (1999). Loss, happiness and postpartum depression: The ultimate paradox. *Canadian Psychology*, 40(2), p. 162–178. https://doi.org/10.1037/h0086834

O'Mahen, H.A., Grieve, H., Jones, J., McGinley, J., Woodford, J., and Wilkinson, E. (2015). Women's experiences of factors affecting treatment engagement and adherence in internet delivered Behavioural Activation for Postnatal Depression. *Internet Interventions*, 2(1), **p.** 84–90.

Raymond, N.C., Pratt, R.J., Godecker, A., Harrison, P.A., Kim, H., Kuendig, J., and O'Brien, J.M. (2014). Addressing perinatal depression in a group of underserved urban women: A focus group study. *BMC Pregnancy Childbirth*, 14, p. 336. https://doi.org/10.1186/1471-2393-14-336

Read, D.M.Y., Crockett, J., and Mason, R. (2012). 'It was a horrible shock': The experience of motherhood and women's family size preferences. *Women's Studies International Forum*, 35, p. 12–21.

Schmied, V., Black, E., Naidoo, N., Dahlen, H.G., and Liamputtong, P. (2017). Migrant women's experiences, meanings and ways of dealing with postnatal depression: A met-ethnographic study. *PLoS One*, 12(3), e0172385. https://doi.org/10.1371/journal.pone.0172385

Staneva, A.A., Bogossian, F., and Wittkowski, A. (2015). The experience of psychological distress, depression, and anxiety during pregnancy: A meta-synthesis of qualitative research. *Midwifery*, 31, p. 563–573. https://doi.org.10.1016/j.midw.2015.03.015

Stone, M., and Kokanovic, M. (2016). 'Halfway towards recovery': Rehabilitating the relational self in narratives of postnatal depression, *Social Science and Medicine*, 163, p. 98–106. https://doi.org/10.1016/j.socscimed.2016.06.040

Tobin, C.L., Di Napoli, P., and Beck, C.T. (2018). Refugee and immigrant women's experiences of postpartum depression: A meta-synthesis. *Journal of Transcultural Nursing*, 29(1), p. 84–100. https://doi.org/10.1177/1043659616686167

Ugarriza, D.N. (2002). Postpartum depressed women's explanation of depression. *Journal of Nursing Scholarship*, 34(3), p. 227–233. https://doi.org/10.1111/j.1547-5069.2002.00227.x

VanderMeulen, H., Strauss, R., Lin, Y. et al. (2020). The contribution of iron deficiency to the risk of peripartum transfusion: A retrospective case control study. *BMC Pregnancy Childbirth*, 20, p. 196. https://doi.org/10.1186/s12884-020-02886-z

Wittkowski, A., Garrett, C., Calam, R., and Weisburg, D. (2017). Self-report measures of parental self-efficacy: A systematic review of the current literature. *Journal of Child and Family Studies*, 26, p. 2960–2978. https://doi.org/10.1007/s10826-017-0830-5

8 Barriers to Treatment
Stigma and Shame Leading to Silence

It is clear that throughout the world, there are significant barriers that stop women from gaining access to treatment for maternal mental illness. In the UK alone, a 2017 survey by the Royal College of Obstetricians and Gynaecologists (Russell et al., 2017) found that only 31% of women had been asked about their mental health by their GP or midwife at their booking-in appointment. In their research into the prevalence of psychiatric disorders during pregnancy in Sweden, Anderson et al. (2003) found that among those women who were diagnosed in pregnancy with a psychiatric or mood disorder, only 5.5% underwent any kind of treatment; either psychophar-macological or psychotherapeutic. This implied that some 95% of women diagnosed with a mental illness in pregnancy received no treatment at all. There would seem to be a substantial lack of recognition of maternal mental illness (Ford et al., 2017; Gavin et al., 2005). Yet, evidence shows that women with depression in pregnancy are far more likely to go on to have postnatal depression (Milgrom et al., 2008; O'Hara & Swain, 1996). Other research also highlights the low percentage of women who receive treatment for postnatal depression (Goodman & Tyer-Viola, 2010; Horowitz & Cousins, 2006). It is plausible that the large proportion of women receiving no treatment suggests the existence of significant barriers preventing access to treatment.

Barriers to treatment are complicated, with multilevel barriers (Sambrook Smith et al., 2019) and include inadequate resourcing of care (Brown et al., 2009); stigma (Bilszta et al., 2010; Goodman, 2009; Myors et al., 2015; O'Mahen & Flynn, 2008); difficulty in expressing feelings due to shame and guilt, as well as negative attitudes which reinforced these feelings, lack of knowledge in healthcare providers (Dadi et al., 2021); confusion about the roles of different care providers within the maternal time-period (Sambrook Smith et al., 2019); lack of sufficient training of midwives and health prac-titioners who are front-line staff and are best placed to offer help and advice (Sambrook Smith et al., 2019); and structural inequalities due to difficulty with transportation to appointment and demands on time (Goodman, 2009), food insecurity, gender-based violence, and lack of education (Howard & Khalifeh, 2020). There also seems to be a deficit in general knowledge of women and their families of maternal mental illness, what it is, what it looks

DOI: 10.4324/9781003154891-9

like and how they can gain help and treatment. In this area, the family can play a significant role in recognising maternal mental illness. Often women do not realise they are unwell, lack insight into their illness and believe their symptoms are 'normal' during pregnancy and the postnatal period. Particularly women with postpartum psychosis who often do not realise the level of distress they are exhibiting to others. There may also be significant cultural differences, as recent research shows that women from ethnic minority backgrounds (Chinese and South Asian, for example) are not cognisant of symptoms and seem unfamiliar with maternal mental health conditions (Sambrook Smith et al., 2019). The group which does seem to be of particularly high risk of developing maternal mental illness is the younger age group of women under 25, who may present with anxiety-related disorders and trauma-related PTSD (Lockwood Estrin et al., 2019).

One important worry for many women is the fear of their baby being removed from their care if they admit to being depressed (Bauer et al., 2014; Boots Family Trust et al., 2013; Dennis & Chung-Lee, 2006). Another concern may be that seeking help from a medical practitioner may result in having to take medication, which can cause anxiety about the detrimental effects on the unborn fetus (Anke, Slinning & Skjelstad, 2019) or passing through breast milk. Other difficulties may also be that there is little care on offer, or the care is quite fragmented, so the healthcare professionals have little to offer other than medication, or do not see this as part of their responsibility (Ford et al., 2019). For those that do access treatment, the compliance rates are often poor, particularly for those taking medication, with higher rates of discontinuation of medication (Munk-Olsen, Gasse & Laursen, 2012; Petersen et al., 2011). Attrition rates in psychological therapies are also high (O'Mahen et al., 2015), and often occur prematurely (Myors et al., 2015), possibly due to the nature and complexity of the perinatal period (O'Mahen et al., 2012). A mixed-methods study into the preferences and concerns of antidepressant usage aimed to highlight possible causal factors, which might explain why so many depressed women failed to engage in treatment within the perinatal period (Battle et al., 2013). This study showed a high comorbidity of anxiety with depression, which supported other studies of a similar nature (Grigoriadis et al., 2011; Wenzel, Gorman & O'Hara, 2001), as well as the role of distress within a woman's relationships (Battle et al., 2013; Beck, 2001; Whisman et al., 2011). There is clearly a difficulty in diagnosis, and this may be due to a perceived sense of stigmatization and shame, rendering women silent, not only with health professionals, but also within their own families (McLoughlin, 2013; Staneva, Bogossian & Wittkowski, 2015). These barriers to treatment are important, as they hinder women firstly asking for treatment, then accessing and continuing treatment at a time when it is vital.

The most significant barriers to treatment, which are cited in much of the research into maternal mental illness are shame, stigma and silence, which are briefly outlined below. In the research, guilt and shame were stated as felt by many women (Beck, 2002; Bennett et al., 2007; Chan, Williamson & McCutcheon, 2009; Coates, Ayers & de Visser, 2014; Knudson-Martin & Silverstein, 2009; Mollard, 2014; Stone & Kokanovic, 2016; Ugarriza, 2002), and was often due to their sense of the stigma of mental illness (Edwards & Timmons, 2005; Staneva et al., 2015; Tobin, Di Napoli & Beck, 2018). This would lead women to hide their illness and to silence themselves (Coates et al., 2014) or to 'wear a mask' (Bennett et al., 2007; Chan et al., 2009).

Stigmatisation

Stigma, the negative attitudes towards and the rejection of those who are mentally ill, has been researched increasingly over recent decades (Byrne, 2001; Masuda & Latzman, 2011; Nosek, Kennedy & Gudmundsdottir, 2010) and is a well-documented barrier to engagement and compliance in treatment (Bates & Stickley, 2013; Vogel et al., 2013). Stigma is also prevalent within perinatal mental health disorders (Goodman, 2009; Mauthner, 2002; McLoughlin, 2013; Myors et al., 2015; O'Mahen & Flynn, 2008; Staneva et al., 2015). Mothers with mental illness say they can experience stigmatisation from society and from within their own families (Bilszta et al., 2010; Davies & Allen, 2007; Di Mascio et al., 2008; Edwards & Timmons, 2005; Hanley & Long, 2006; Holopainen, 2002; Krumm & Becker, 2006). This causes them to become hesitant in revealing their inability to cope, due to the shame they feel from admitting their 'weakness'. Mantle (2002) states that the reason postnatal depression continues to go undetected and untreated is due to stigmatisation.

Shame

For Gabor Maté, shame is one of the deepest of our emotions and due to the negativity produced by it, we are likely to do as much as we possibly can in order to avoid it (2019).

DeYoung (2015) approaches shame from a relational and neurobiological perspective and believes that shame is actually physical, that it hurts and that the pain of shame can be unbearable. In her research on shame, she discovered that people push it away as fast as possible and cover it with more tolerable states of being. However, when a person covers their shame, they are actually compensating, by using masks, or '*sleights of mind*' (DeYoung, 2015). Those people are pretending to be something or someone that they are not. DeYoung (2015) believes that people do this because they believe that there is actually something wrong with them: '*Shame is an experience of one's felt sense of self disintegrating in relation to a dysregulating other*' (DeYoung, 2015, p xiii).

By using the term, 'dysregulating other' DeYoung (2015) implies that shame is a relational experience. She believes it does not happen to a person alone, it depends upon the 'other' who responds in a negative way, causing the human psyche to feel an intense, unpleasant experience of non-acceptance. This, she believes, can cause the psyche to fragment. This experience of self as mis-attuned to, or mis-attuning may cause humans to believe things about themselves that are faulty or not real. It is shame about self that causes a human to cover up or mask their real self. Heller and LaPierre (2012) show how early trauma, such as feeling unwelcomed, rejected, unlovable, bad, wrong and sometimes not quite human gives rise to conscious and unconscious shame-based identification (p. 125). For women in the perinatal period, this is of primary importance, because the infant of a mother with mental illness could grow up to feel rejected, unlovable, bad or wrong, because of the mother's significant ill-health.

DeYoung (2015) sees shame as a relational trauma which engenders self-protection mechanisms within the person, such as impaired capacity for connection (Heller & LaPierre, 2012). Brown (2007) calls shame the '*Silent Epidemic*' (p. xvii) and states that it unravels our connection to others. She calls shame '*the fear of disconnection – the fear of being perceived as flawed and unworthy of acceptance or belonging*' (p. xxv). Shame causes humans to pretend to be something they are not. Buultjens & Liamputtong (2007) highlight this in perinatal mental illness: '*Sadly, many women go undetected and suffer in silence for fear of disapproval and rejection*' (p. 87). McIntosh (1993) concluded that women who felt shame chose not to seek help, which was corroborated within research from Bilszta et al. (2010), and Holopainen (2002). Women with traumatic backgrounds particularly felt shame (Talbot & Gamble, 2008). Women also avoided seeking help until the depression became debilitating (McIntosh, 1993). Shame may cause women to pretend to be okay, when in fact, they are extremely unwell. Some women report of refusing to speak to healthcare professionals about their symptoms for fear of being labelled mad. This should be a concern for those working within the NHS and aligns with the findings of qualitative studies which found a lack of training and knowledge within mental health professionals, GPs, midwives and health visitors (Button et al., 2017; Byatt et al., 2013; Foulkes, 2011; Jarrett, 2016; O'Mahen et al., 2015; O'Mahony et al., 2012; Nakku et al., 2016; Slade et al., 2010). There is a need for consistent and thorough training and education among health care providers, particularly those working within mental health regarding shame and how to mitigate this experience effectively. It is important to eradicate stereotyping and outdated views and behaviour which should not be acceptable within any healthcare system.

Silence – The consequence of stigma and shame in perinatal mental illness

Silence is a fundamental part of maternal mental illness. Women with such mental illness say they find themselves on the margins of society. Many feminists write about women's voices being silenced as a result of their experiences within a patriarchal society (Belenky et al., 1986; Brown & Gilligan, 1992;

Jack & Ali, 2010). Silence contributes to the length of time women take to seek help. Mauthner (1999) states: '*Postpartum depression occurs when women are unable to experience, express and validate their feelings and needs within supportive, accepting and non-judgmental interpersonal relationships and cultural context*' (p. 160). In much of the research literature on maternal mental illness, silence is a significant problem, with women silencing themselves due to stigma, shame, guilt and embarrassment as well as due to a fear of losing their infant (Boots Family Trust Alliance et al., 2013; Buultjens & Liamputtong, 2007; Tobin et al., 2018). Silence is a prevalent feature of maternal mental illness and a compounding problem for diagnosis.

Jack (1991, 1999) wrote an influential model on silencing the self (STS) after a longitudinal study of the description of the experience of clinically depressed women. These women detailed how they actively silenced themselves in order to maintain their relationships, to maintain their own physical or psychological safety and also to avoid conflict (Jack, 1991, 1999, 2003). She found that this self-silencing was in fact a deeply cultural process, which led to women feeling a loss of self, and feeling lost within their own lives. The narrative from Jack's research was of silencing self, due to depression caused by a sense of norms, prescribed values, and images of how women should be, from a male-centred world, leading these women into a position of shame, desperation, and anger from their sense of entrapment and self-betrayal. As silence is such a fundamental part of perinatal distress, it seems plausible that there may be a similar form of self-silencing occurring. Jack uses many aspects of psychological theories – attachment theory, relational theory, and cognitive theory, to substantiate her argument of the vulnerability of women to depression, through a lack of intimacy (1991, 1999). Disconnection and isolation, again language that is used in perinatal distress, were precipitating and maintaining factors in her work on depression. She highlights the interconnectedness of personal, cognitive, social, and biological, and the particular threat relational disconnection constitutes to the self, helping to show how relational disconnectedness, mother to infant, may also exacerbate perinatal mental illness, and increase an infant's susceptibility to life-long mental illness. Staneva et al. (2015), in their meta-synthesis of qualitative research, support this concept of self-silencing, particularly if the woman felt isolated or misunderstood by their partner. This silence then had a profound impact on the woman's emotional state through pregnancy, birth and postnatally.

The mother-infant bond is one of the most intimate bonds within humans and is now shown to be crucial to the development of the infant's brain and sense of identity (Schore, 2003). It is possible that this lack of bond, inability to bond, or a mother's perceived lack of bond with their baby reinforces and heightens the mother's sense of mental illness. If the mother was not mothered herself due to her own mother being unwell in the perinatal period, a system of trans-generational scripting may have passed from grandmother to mother and could now be passed onto the infant. Within Transactional

Analysis, this is identified within the theory of trans-generational trauma (Noriega Gayol, 2004), which identifies how scripts could be handed down from one generation to the next, for example, alcoholism (p. 312) and possibly perinatal mental illness. Advances in neuroscience and epigenetics are beginning to scientifically suggest the mechanisms for this passing down through the generations of illness and affective states. Yet they are both still in their infancy and conclusions might thus be premature.

Within their meta-synthesis of qualitative studies on depression, anxiety and distress in pregnancy, Staneva et al. (2015) believe women silence their voices and themselves in their relationships both intimately and socially due to their experiences of powerlessness. They found that women who felt misunderstood by their partners felt alone or lacked resources and support and chose to remain silent. Those who remained silent seemed to have difficulties developing an attachment to their babies, and a more profound level of postnatal depression (Staneva et al., 2015). In their qualitative systematic review on postpartum depression help-seeking barriers, Dennis and Chung-Lee (2006) found that women from culturally diverse backgrounds did not proactively seek help for their illness and stayed silent. This silence is a problem for treatment. If women stay silent and feel unable to admit to their distress and discount or minimise their illness, then this silence may contribute to the lack of diagnosis and treatment of this condition (Dennis & Chung-Lee, 2006).

Shame within treatment

In psychotherapy, when treating maternal mental illness, it is very easy to shame a woman, particularly if we are sharing information about the damage that may be caused to an infant through poor maternal attachment, yet not even realise this is what is happening in the moment. So often, women are hypersensitive to anything they detect that might signify they are not doing a 'good enough' job. One way to notice that something is shaming is the silence that then may occur. That silence can be absolutely deafening. Women are struggling already and are distressed by what they perceive to be their own inadequacies as a parent. Well-intentioned psychoeducation may not in fact be helpful at all, particularly at the outset of therapy. It is also really important to be aware of any interpretations that are made. These are our own subjective views of reality and may bear no resemblance to that of the woman in front of us. What is more important is a level of what Safran and Muran call 'meta-communication' (2000). Countertransference disclosure is important in therapy, and some elements of self-disclosure will occur through the need to articulate our sense of what may be going on in the moment. However, discretion needs to be used. I like to think carefully whether what I am about to say is for the client's benefit, or actually my own. If it is for my own, then I have learnt over time to be careful to pause and possibly not speak, to remain curious and observing, to see what may transpire. I like to hold the need to explore lightly, to be tentative about my curiosity and exploration. This is not to say that I do not challenge. I do. However, I try to always remain mindful about the challenge, and to remain within an exploratory framework, rather than something that might feel concretising to my client. It is also important to remain in a collaborative state with our clients, to help them to self-reflect and to explore their own subjectivity, as well as to explore ours. Safran and Muran talk about Christopher Bollas' idea of therapists 'announcing their subjectivity' (2000). I believe this then frees the client up to tell me whether I am right or wrong, and it reminds me not to assume that I am right. This is important in the sense of open communication and mutuality in relationship. I am trying to engender as close to equality of the power dynamic with my client, even though I understand that they may always place me in the position of power or knowledge. Actually, they are the expert of their own self, not me. I can suppose, be curious, be mindful, and be subjective, but I cannot be definitive. If I am wrong, which I often am, then it is important also for me to accept that I am wrong, and to help the client to put me right. This is about the therapist taking responsibility for their actions, another element from metacommunication that Safran and Muran define. When my client and I have a rupture, which is absolutely inevitable within psychotherapy, then my role is to take responsibility for my part in the rupture, to apologise, if necessary, and to work with the client, collaboratively, so that we can forge a new experience of repairing the rupture. This may never have happened before as she may be expecting the rupture to go unrepaired, and for her to remain dysregulated, as she was before.

A final thing to say at this point is that we will also go to the same place over and over again, finding the same point of stuckness. This is important. Not only is this a way of discovering how deep the impasse is, but it is also helpful in showing movement in the therapy, and the level of success the client may feel. Being stuck does not mean that the therapy is a failure. It does mean that the therapy needs to keep going for a while longer, and that the impasse is maybe held at a deeper level which neither therapist nor client yet understands. I talk more about this in the section on treatment.

References

Anderson, L., Sundström-Poromaa, I., Bixo, M., Wulff, M., Bondestam, K., and Aström, M. (2003). Point prevalence of psychiatric disorders during the second trimester of pregnancy: A population-based study. *American Journal of Obstetrics & Gynecology*, 189, p. 148–154. https://doi.org/10.1067/mob.2003.336

Anke, T.M.S., Slinning, K., and Skjelstad, D.V. (2019). "What if I get ill?" Perinatal concerns and preparations in primi- and multiparous women with bipolar disorder. *International Journal of Bipolar Disorders*, 7, Article 7. https://doi.org/10.1186/s40345-019-0143-2

Bates, L., and Stickley, T. (2013). Confronting Goffman: How can mental health nurses effectively challenge stigma? A critical review of the literature. *Journal of Psychiatric and Mental Health Nursing*, 20, p. 269–575. https://doi.org/10.1111/j.1365-2850.2012.01957.x

Battle, C.L., Salisbury, A.L., Schofield, C.A., and Ortiz-Hernandez, S. (2013). Perinatal antidepressant use: Understanding women's preferences and concerns. *Journal of Psychiatric Practice*, 19(6), p. 443–453. https://doi.org/10.1097/01. pra.0000438183.74359.46

Bauer, A., Parsonage, M., Knapp, M., Iemmi, V., and Adelaja, B. (2014). *Costs of Perinatal Mental Health Problems*. Centre for Mental Health. Retrieved from https://www. centreformentalhealth.org.uk/publications/costs-perinatal-mental-health-problems [accessed 21.11.21].

Beck, C.T. (2001). Predictors of postpartum depression: An update. *Nursing Research*, 50(5), p. 275–285. https://doi.org/10.1097/00006199-200109000-00004

Beck, C.T. (2002). Postpartum depression: A metasynthesis. *Qualitative Health Research*, 12, p. 469–488. https://doi.org/10.1177/104973202129120016

Belenky, M.F., Clinchy, B.M., Goldberger, N.R., and Tarule, J.M. (1986). *Women's Ways of Knowing: The Development of Self, Voice, and Mind*. New York: Basic Books.

Bennett, H., Boon, H., Romans, S., and Grootendorst, P. (2007). Becoming the best mom that I can: women's experiences of managing depression during pregnancy – A qualitative study. *BMC Women's Health*, 7, p. 13. https://doi.org/10.1186/1472-6874-7-13

Bilszta, J., Ericksen, J., Buist, A., and Milgrom, J. (2010). Women's experiences of postnatal depression – Beliefs and attitudes as barriers to care. *Australian Journal of Advanced Nursing*, 27(3), p. 44–54. Corpus ID: 44990132.

Boots Family Trust Alliance, Netmums, Institute of Health Visiting, Tommy's, The Royal College of Midwives (2013). *Perinatal Mental Health Experiences of Women and Health Professionals*. London: Boots Family Trust.

Brown, B. (2007). *I Thought It Was Just Me (But It Isn't) – Making the Journey from "What Will People Think?" to "I Am Enough"*. New York: Avery.

Brown, L.M., and Gilligan, C. (1992). *Meeting at the Crossroads: Women's Psychology and Girls' Development*. Cambridge, MA: Harvard University Press.

Brown, M., Mills, N., McCalmont, C., and Lees, S. (2009). Perinatal mental health services. *Primary Health Care*, 19(8), p. 36–39. http://primaryhealthcare.rcnpublishing. co.uk/archive/article-perinatal-mental-health-services

Button, S., Lee, S., Shakespeare, J., and Ayers, S. (2017). Seeking help for perinatal psychological distress: A meta-synthesis of women's experiences. *The British Journal of General Practice*, 67(663), p. e692–e699. https://doi.org/10.3399/bjgp17X692549

Buultjens, M., and Liamputtong, P. (2007). When giving life starts to take the life out of you: women's experiences of depression after childbirth. *Midwifery*, 23(1), p. 77–91. https://doi.org/10.1016/j.midw.2006.04.002

Byatt, N., Biebel, K., Friedman, L., Debordes-Jackson, G., Ziedonis, D., and Pbert, L. (2013). Patients' views on depression care in obstetric settings: How do they compare to the views of perinatal health care professionals? *General Hospital Psychiatry*, 35(6), p. 598–604. https://doi.org/10.1016/j.genhosppsych.2013.07.011

Byrne, P. (2001). Psychiatric stigma. *The British Journal of Psychiatry*, 178, p. 281–284. https://doi.org/10.1192/bjp.178.3.281

Chan, S.W., Williamson, V., and McCutcheon, H. (2009). A comparative study of the experiences of a group of Hong Kong Chinese women and Australian women diagnosed with postnatal depression. *Perspectives in Psychiatric Care*, 45(2), p. 108–118. https://doi.org/10.1111/j.1744-6163.2009.00211.x

Coates, R., Ayers, S., and de Visser, R. (2014). Women's experiences of postnatal distress: A qualitative study. *BMC Pregnancy & Childbirth*, 14, p. 359. https://doi. org/10.1186/1471-2393-14-359

Dadi, A.F., Miller, E.R., Azale, T., and Mwanri, L. (2021). "We do not know how to screen and provide treatment": A qualitative study of barriers and enablers of implementing perinatal depression health services in Ethiopia. *International Journal of Mental Health Systems*, 2021 May 5, 15(1), p. 41. https://doi.org/10.1186/s13033-021-00466-y PMID: 33952338; PMCID: PMC8098000.

Davies, B., and Allen, D. (2007). Integrating 'mental illness' and 'motherhood': The positive use of surveillance by health professionals. A qualitative study. *International Journal of Nursing Studies*, 44(3), p. 365–376. https://doi.org/10.1016/j.ijnurstu.2005.11.033

Dennis, C.-L., and Chung-Lee, L. (2006). Postpartum depression help-seeking barriers and maternal treatment preferences: A qualitative systematic review. *Birth*, 33, p. 323–331. https://doi.org/10.1111/j.1523-536X.2006.00130.x

DeYoung, P. (2015). *Understanding and Treating Chronic Shame – A Relational/Neurobiological Approach*. New York and Hove: Routledge.

Edwards, E., and Timmons, S. (2005). A qualitative study of stigma among women suffering postnatal illness. *Journal of Mental Health*, 14(5), p. 471–481. https://doi.org/10.1080/09638230500271097

Ford, E., Roomi, H., Hugh, H., and van Marwijk, H. (2019). Understanding barriers to women seeking and receiving help for perinatal mental health problems in UK general practice: Development of a questionnaire. *Primary Health Care Research & Development*, Dec 12, (20), p. e156. https://doi.org/10.1017/S1463423619000902. PMID: 31826794; PMCID: PMC7003527.

Ford, E., Shakespeare, J., Elias, F., and Ayers, S. (2017). Recognition and management of perinatal depression and anxiety by general practitioners: A systematic review. *Family Practice*, 34(1), p. 11–19. https://doi.org/10.1093/fampra/cmw101. Epub 2016 Sep 22. PMID: 27660558.

Foulkes, M. (2011). Enablers and barriers to seeking help for a postpartum mood disorder. *Journal of Obstetric, Gynecologic & Neonatal Nursing*, 40(4), p. 450–457. https://doi.org/10.14288/1.0132692

Gavin, N.I., Gaynes, B.N., Lohr, K.N., Meltzer-Brody, S., Gartlehner, G., and Swinson, T. (2005). Perinatal depression: A systematic review of prevalence and incidence. *Obstetrics & Gynecology*, 106(5), p. 1071–1083. https://doi.org/10.1097/01.AOG.0000183597.31630.db

Goodman, J.H. (2009). Women's attitudes, preferences, and perceived barriers to treatment for perinatal depression. *Birth*, 36(1), p. 60–69. https://doi.org/10.1111/j.1523-536X.2008.00296.x

Goodman, J.H., and Tyer-Viola, L. (2010). Detection, treatment and referral of perinatal depression and anxiety by obstetrical providers. *Journal of Women's Health*, 19(3), p. 477–490. https://doi.org/10.1089/jwh.2008.1352

Grigoriadis, S., de Camps Meschino, D., Barrons, E., Bradley, L., Eady, A., Fishell, A., Mamisachvili, L., Cook, G.S., O'Keefe, M., Romans, S., and Ross, L.E. (2011). Mood and anxiety disorders in a sample of Canadian perinatal women referred for psychiatric care. *Archive of Women's Mental Health*, 14(4), p. 325–333. https://doi.org/10.1007/s00737-011-0223-5

Hanley, J., and Long, B. 2006. A study of Welsh mothers' experiences of postnatal depression. *Midwifery*, 22(2), p. 147–157. https://doi.org/10.1016/j.midw.2005.08.004

Heller, L., and LaPierre, A. (2012). *Healing Developmental Trauma: How Early Trauma Affects Self-Regulation, Self-Image, and the Capacity for Relationship*. Berkeley, CA: North Atlantic Books.

Holopainen, D. (2002). The experience of seeking help for postnatal depression. *Advanced Journal of Nursing*, 19, p. 39–44. https://doi.org/10.1054/midw.2001.0259

Horowitz, J.A., and Cousins, A. (2006). Postpartum depression treatment rates for at-risk women. *Nursing Research*, 55(2), p. s23–s27. https://doi.org/10.1097/00006199-200603001-00005

Howard, L., and Khalifeh, H. (2020). Perinatal mental health: A review of progress and challenges. *World Psychiatry*, 19(3), p. 313–327. https://doi.org/10.1002/wps.20769

Jack, D.C. (1991). *Silencing the Self: Women and Depression*. Cambridge, MA: Harvard University Press.

Jack, D.C. (1999). Silencing the self: Inner dialogues and outer realities. In T.E. Joiner & J.C. Coyne (Eds), *The Interactional Nature of Depression: Advances in Interpersonal Approaches*. pp. 221–246. Washington, DC: American Psychological Association.

Jack, D.C. (2003). The anger of hope and the anger of despair: How anger relates to women's depression. In J. Stoppard & L. McMullen (Eds), *Situating Sadness: Women and Depression in Social Context*. pp. 62–87. New York University Press Series on Qualitative Studies in Psychology, Michelle Fine and Jeanne Maracek (Series Eds). New York: New York University Press.

Jack, D.C., and Ali, A. (Eds) (2010). *Silencing the Self Across Cultures: Depression and Gender in the Social World*. New York: Oxford University Press.

Jarrett, P.M. (2016). Pregnant women's experiences of depression care. *The Journal of Mental Health Training, Education & Practice*, 11(1), p. 33–47. https://doi.org/10.1108/JMHTEP-05-2015-0023

Knudson-Martin, C., and Silverstein, R. (2009). Suffering in silence: A qualitative meta-data-analysis of postpartum depression. *Journal of Marital and Family Therapy*, 35(2), p. 145–158. https://doi.org/10.1111/j.1752-0606.2009.00112.x

Krumm, S., and Becker, T. (2006). Subjective views of motherhood in women with mental illness – A sociological perspective. *Journal of Mental Health*, 15(4), p. 449–460. https://doi.org/10.1080/09638230600801470

Lockwood Estrin, G., Ryan, E., Trevillion, K., Demilew, J., Bick, D., Pickles, A., and Howard, L. (2019). Young pregnant women and risk for mental disorders: Findings from an early pregnancy cohort. *British Journal of Psychiatry Open*, 5(2), E21. https://doi.org/10.1192/bjo.2019.6

Mantle, F. (2002). The role of alternative medicine in treating postnatal depression. *Complementary Therapies in Nursing and Midwifery*, 8, p. 197–203. https://doi.org/10.1054/ctnm.2002.0647

Masuda, A., and Latzman, R.D. (2011). Examining associations among factor-analytically derived components of mental health stigma, distress, and psychological flexibility. *Personality and Individual Differences*, 51(4), p. 435–438. https://doi.org/10.1016/j.paid.2011.04.008

Maté, G. (2019). *When the Body Says No: The Cost of Hidden Stress*. London, UK: Vermillion.

Mauthner, N. (1999). Feeling low and feeling really bad about feeling low: Women's experiences of motherhood and postpartum depression. *Canadian Psychology*, 40, p. 143–161.

Mauthner, N.S. (2002). *The Darkest Days of My Life: Stories of Postpartum Depression*. Cambridge, MA: Harvard University Press.

McIntosh, J. (1993). Postpartum depression: Women's help-seeking behavior and perceptions of cause. *Journal of Advanced Nursing*, 18, p. 178–184. https://doi.org/10.1046/j.1365-2648-1993.18020178.x

McLoughlin, J. (2013). Stigma associated with postnatal depression: A literature review. *British Journal of Midwifery*, 21(11). https://doi.org/10.12968/bjom.2013.21.11.784

Milgrom, J., Gemmill, A.W., Bilszta, J.A., Hayes, B., Barnett, B., Brooks, J., Ericksen, J., Ellwood, D., and Buist, A. (2008). Antenatal risk factors for postnatal depression: A large prospective study. *Journal of Affective Disorders*, 108, p. 147–157. https://doi.org/10.1016/j.jad.2007.10.014

Mollard, E.K. (2014). A qualitative meta-synthesis and theory of postpartum depression. *Issues in Mental Health Nursing*, 35(9), p. 656–663. https://doi.org/10.3109/01612840.2014.893044

Munk-Olsen, T., Gasse, C., and Laursen, T.M. (2012). Prevalence of antidepressant use and contacts with psychiatrists and psychologists in pregnant and postpartum women. *Acta Psychiatrica Scandinavica*, 125(4), p. 318–324. https://doi.org/10.1111/j.1600-0447.2011.01784.x

Myors, K.A., Johnson, M., Cleary, M., and Schmied, V. (2015). Engaging women at risk for poor perinatal mental health outcomes: A mixed-methods study. *International Journal of Mental Health Nursing*, 24, p. 241–252. https://doi.org/10.1111/inm.12109

Nakku, J.E.M., Okello, E.S., Honikman, D.K.S., Ssebunnya, J., Ndyanabangi, S., Hanlon, C., and Kigozi, F. (2016). Perinatal mental health care in a rural African district, Uganda: A qualitative study of barriers, facilitators and needs. *BMC Health Services Research,* 16, p. 295. https://doi.org/10.1186/s12913-016-1547-7

Noriega Gayol, G. (2004). Codependence: A transgenerational script. *Transactional Analysis Journal*, 34(4), p. 312–322. https://doi.org/10.1177/036215370403400404

Nosek, M.P., Kennedy, H.P., and Gudmundsdottir, M.P. (2010). Silence, stigma, and shame: A postmodern analysis of distress during the menopause. *Advances in Nursing Science*, 33(3), p. e24–e36. https://doi.org/10.1097/ANS.0b013e3181eb41e8

O'Hara, M.W., and Swain, A.M., (1996). Rates and risk of postpartum depression: A meta-analysis. *International Review of Psychiatry*, 8, p. 37–54. https://doi.org/10.3109/09540269609037816

O'Mahen, H., Fedock, G., Henshaw, E., Himle, J.A., Forman, J., and Flynn, H.A. (2012). Modifying CBT for perinatal depression: What do women want? A qualitative study. *Cognitive and Behavioural Practice*, 19(2), p. 359–371. https://doi.org/10.1016/j.cbpra.2011.05.005

O'Mahen, H.A., and Flynn, H.A. (2008). Preferences and perceived barriers to treatment for depression during the perinatal period. *Journal of Women's Health*, 17(8), p. 1301–1309. https://doi.org/10.1089/jwh.2007.0631

O'Mahen, H.A., Grieve, H., Jones, J., McGinley, J., Woodford, J., and Wilkinson, E. (2015). Women's experiences of factors affecting treatment engagement and adherence in internet delivered behavioural activation for postnatal depression. *Internet Interventions,* 2(1), p. 84–90. https://doi.org/10.1016/j.invent.2014.11.003

O'Mahony, J.M., Donnelly, T.T., Bouchal, S.R., and Est, D. (2012). Barriers and facilitators of social supports for immigrant and refugee women coping with postpartum depression. *Advances in Nursing Science*, 35(3), p. e42–56. https://doi.org/10.1097/ANS.0b013e3182626137

Petersen, I., Gilbert, R.E., Evans, S.J., Man, S.L., and Nazareth, I. (2011). Pregnancy as a major determinant for discontinuation of antidepressants: An analysis of data from the health improvement network. *Journal of Clinical Psychiatry*, 72, p. 979–985. https://doi.org/10.4088/JCP.10m06090blu

Russell, K., Ashley, A., Chan, G., Givson, S., and Jones, R. (2017). *Maternal Mental Health – Women's Voices*. London, England: Royal College of Obstetricians and Gynaecologists.

Safran, J.D., and Muran, J.C. (2000). *Negotiating the Therapeutic Alliance: A Relational Treatment Guide*. New York: Guildford Press.

Sambrook Smith, M., Lawrence, V., Sadler, E., and Easter, A. (2019). Barriers to accessing mental health services for women with perinatal mental illness: Systematic review and meta-synthesis of qualitative studies in the UK. *BMJ Open*, 9(1), e024803. https://doi.org/10.1136/bmjopen-2018-024803

Schore, A.N. (2003). *Affect Regulation and the Repair of the Self*. London: W.W. Norton.

Slade, P., Morrell, C.J., Rigby, A., Ricci, K., Spittlehouse, J., and Brugha, T.S. (2010). Postnatal women's experiences of management of depressive symptoms: A qualitative study. *British Journal of General Practice*, 60(580), p. e440–448. https://doi.org/10.3399/bjgp10X532611

Staneva, A.A., Bogossian, F., and Wittkowski, A. (2015). The experience of psychological distress, depression, and anxiety during pregnancy: A meta-synthesis of qualitative research. *Midwifery*, 31, p. 563–573. https://doi.org.10.1016/j.midw.2015.03.015

Stone, M., and Kokanovic, M. (2016). 'Halfway towards recovery': Rehabilitating the relational self in narratives of postnatal depression. *Social Science and Medicine*, 163, p. 98–106. https://doi.org/10.1016/j.socscimed.2016.06.040

Talbot, N.L., and Gamble, S.A. (2008). IPT for women with trauma histories in community mental health care. *Journal of Contemporary Psychotherapy*, 38, p. 35–44. https://doi.org.10.1007/s10879-007-9066-9

Tobin, C.L., Di Napoli, P., and Beck, C.T. (2018). Refugee and immigrant Women's experiences of postpartum depression: A meta-synthesis. *Journal of Transcultural Nursing*, 29(1), p. 84–100. https://doi.org/10.1177/1043659616686167

Ugarriza, D.N. (2002). Postpartum depressed women's explanation of depression. *Journal of Nursing Scholarship*, 34(3), p. 277–233. https://doi.org/10.1111/j.1547-5069.2002.00227.x

Vogel, D.L., Bitman, R.L., Hammer, J.H., and Wade, N.G. (2013). Is stigma internalized? The longitudinal impact of public stigma on self-stigma. *Journal of Counseling Psychology*, 60(2), p. 311–316. https://doi.org/10.1037/a0031889

Wenzel, A., Gorman, L., and O'Hara, M.W. (2001). The occurrence of panic and obsessive compulsive symptoms in women with post-partum dysphoria: A prospective study. *Archives of Women's Mental Health*, 4, p. 5–12. https://doi.org/10.1007/s007370170002

Whisman, M.A., Davila, J., and Goodman, S.H. (2011). Relationship adjustment, depression, and anxiety during pregnancy and the postpartum period. *Journal of Family Psychology*, 25(3), p. 375–383. https://doi.org/10.1037/a0023790

Part II

Listening Beyond Words

9   A Relational Approach

Humans are relational creatures. How we think, feel and behave is directly related to our interpersonal relationships (past and present) with other humans. These relationships, from early infancy through to present day, can have a direct impact on our emotional well-being, particularly if we struggle to maintain supportive, healthy relationships and find ourselves in deeply distressing patterns of dysfunctional relating. Everything we do in life is formed through our experience of self with other. No matter what element – political, social, familial, work-related – we are continuously formed and re-formed through our relationships and the way we interact with others. Having good connections with others around us helps us to feel good.

From the moment of conception, pregnant women are in a relationship with their fetus. For some, this relationship may form even prior to conception, particularly if there was a difficulty in conception or the baby has been conceived through artificial reproductive techniques (ART) such as in vitro fertilization (IVF). Many women fantasise about their baby, prior to pregnancy, such as what the baby will look like, or who they will take after, how life will be, and what the family will be like together. Pregnant mothers often talk to or sing to their unborn babies, and many women give their baby significance, believing that the baby is already a thinking, feeling being. The partner may also play a role, relating to their unborn child, listening to its heartbeat, feeling its movement and conferring status to this baby. The couple together make plans and dreams of life after the baby is born. This is such an important part of connection, even prior to conception. We may believe that these fantasies will always be positive. This is not the case at all, as it is dependent upon how the baby was conceived. For example, was conception within a highly functioning relationship at a time that is convenient, or at the opposite extreme, through abuse, rape or when the family is experiencing hardship or fleeing from war. Perhaps, the family cannot afford another mouth to feed, or there is turmoil and unrest within the area they live. All of these elements influence the fantasies.

This relationship between mother and infant continues through birth and life, until there is a rupture, in whatever form that may take – physical, with the death of the mother or child, or emotional/psychological, with the death

DOI: 10.4324/9781003154891-11

of the relationship. This relationship is of absolute primary importance to the survival of the infant, and the survival of the human species. Yet, a woman experiencing maternal mental illness may be struggling with this aspect. It may even be the baby itself that is seen as the cause of her difficulties, particularly if the birth was highly traumatic. Other concerns may be worry that she has not bonded with her baby in the way she feels she should have, or that society dictates. She may feel dread at the birth, or indeed at the baby itself, if she feels that the baby has a role to play in her illness. She may wonder how she will cope, or already not be coping. She may feel traumatised by the pregnancy, the birth or is overwhelmed by the responsibility of having a child, knowing this will continue for many years. She may be concerned that her lack as a parent, inability to cope, or sense of engulfment in responsibility, may harm her child and set them up for a lifetime of mental illness, passed trans-generationally from mother to child. She might intensely fear she will be the cause of her child's future negative behavioural traits, knowing that during pregnancy and the first two crucial years, she was riddled with anxiety, fear, numbness and a sense of hopelessness as a mother. Therefore, it makes sense to me that the way to help and to heal is through the relationship, helping to forge a good enough relationship between therapist and client, as a model for the woman to draw on in her relationship with her baby.

The transition to motherhood can be wrought with difficult feelings, myths, naivety and foreboding, no matter how well-grounded the mother is, or how much the baby is wanted. Often there are also huge cultural, societal and familial expectations about the birth and baby which may place further demands on the mother and her partner to raise their child in the way that is accepted or acceptable, placing added pressure on intimate relationships. Therefore, it makes sense to focus treatment on these relationships, bringing any dysfunctionality to light and exploring where the difficulties may come from. It is also useful to explore the woman's relationship with her mother and her own birth story. Sometimes, these stories of maternal mental illness are transgenerational, a grandmother with a history of bipolar disorder perhaps, or a mother who was also under the care of a mother and baby inpatient psychiatric unit. Nearly always, these stories are ones where relationships have been a struggle. Then add in lack of sleep, exhaustion, emotion, fear, intense responsibility and hormonal fluctuations and these can begin to form a perfect storm of illness.

Storytelling as a part of the therapeutic process

Narrating our distress to another, as part of relational psychotherapy, is fundamental in our pathway to change. Storytelling is age old within humanity: '*Humans are storytellers. It is our nature to make up stories, to interpret everything we perceive. Without awareness, we give our personal power to the story and the story writes itself. With awareness, we recover the control of our story. We see we are the authors and if we don't like our story, we change it*' (Ruiz, 1997). This is how history has been passed down generationally. We also give illness a voice, through the narrative account. This is something I believe is vital in treating women with this illness. Research shows that women silence themselves, and feel silenced by their illness, their family, society and the medical profession. Psychotherapy gives women a voice, as the therapist, we become the witnessing 'other', seeing and hearing the client's distress, their reality and their difficulty. Clients will often tell the same story many times over. This is an opportunity to listen to them, to really hear, and feel what it is like to have their struggle and offers an opportunity to gain a deep understanding of the uniqueness of their story. It also helps me to gauge whether the therapy is effective. When the story begins to shift and change, it is a clue that the client is shifting and changing.

Specificity of treatment

Relational psychotherapy provides a therapeutic frame to work with women through this sometimes difficult and disturbing transition to motherhood. It highlights not only the importance of uncertainty but also curiosity and creativity, and hopes to enhance a woman's ability to engage, attach and bond with her baby. Many women speak of their struggle to gain any kind of treatment for their distress through their doctor or medical service and are often only offered medication. Psychotherapy offers something different to medication giving choice, although this is limited at present by a woman's capacity to fund it, as it is, as yet, rarely funded through health services. Until psychotherapy becomes better known as a suitable and viable treatment and gains government funding, it will remain on the margins, only afforded by those with the available resources.

Yet, relational psychotherapy is particularly useful and valuable in different ways such as:

- Increasing a women's understanding of her distress
- Highlighting the importance and value of the mother/infant bond
- Highlighting the importance of conscious and non-conscious patterns of relating and experience
- Highlighting the importance of the relationship and its co-creative nature
- The importance of the mother/father/caregiver in modelling behaviour both explicitly and implicitly within the parent/infant bond
- Going back into the past to highlight trans-generational patterns of relating within the woman's family, to see if this holds clues to the present difficulties

In research studies, many women state their preference for psychotherapy as a treatment, rather than medication such as antidepressants (Battle et al., 2013; Dennis & Chung-Lee, 2006; Goodman, 2009; O'Mahen & Flynn, 2008;

Pearlstein et al., 2006). In the UK particularly, psychotherapy is rarely offered within the NHS, although some forms of it are offered through something called the 'Improving Access to Psychological Therapies' (IAPT) service. However, recommendations have been made to tailor this support (Department of Health, 2013) and certainly treatment needs to account for the specific nature of illness each woman experiences. O'Mahen et al. (2015) suggest that perinatal-specific treatment, and in particular relevance, is an important factor in bringing women into treatment and keeping them in it. This specificity is a factor that cannot be addressed well with manualised treatment programmes, as they tend to be structured to a specific weekly programme, rather than to the specific nature of each woman's experience. Any kind of large-scale treatment programme will need to address this specificity, if it is to be useful.

Relational psychotherapy

Fowlie and Sills explain relational psychotherapy as bringing '*the psychoanalytic world's rigorous attention to the non-conscious inner world of implicit knowing and relating, together with the humanistic recognition that human being exist in relationship and that real connection with another is the source of well-being and growth*' (2011, p. xxviii). In order to understand relational psychotherapy more fully, it is helpful for us to take a step back to psychotherapy first. 'Psychological therapy' is a generic term in everyday parlance used to describe treatment to improve psychological functioning, or to help with particular behaviour, which is seen as unhelpful, troubling or unusual. This is different to medical treatments, such as pharmacotherapy (e.g. drug treatment) which seek to act on a 'medical disease'. The term 'psychotherapy' covers a wide range of different modalities and styles, such as Cognitive Behavioural Therapy (CBT), Interpersonal Therapy (IPT), Psychoanalysis and Person-Centred Therapy, and its premise is to offer treatment for any form of mental illness. There are all sorts of different ways psychotherapy may be offered, such as one-to-one sessions, for couples, for families and within group settings. Psychotherapy is a form of 'talking therapy', yet this does not give a true picture as there are all sorts of techniques used, such as using creativity, the arts, dance or theatre to explore people's emotional struggles. Consideration of specificity in treatment for mental illness is important. Kwan, Dimidjian and Rizvi (2010) showed that people who received their treatment of choice for particularly depression were more likely to begin their treatment, stay engaged, and continue to attend treatment appointments. As you may imagine, this engagement had a positive impact on the therapeutic alliance and this alliance was a fundamental factor in whether treatment was successful or not (see Chapter 13 for further research on the importance of the therapeutic alliance as a factor in treatment success).

When a client enters psychotherapy, one role the therapist has is to facilitate understanding of whatever it is they are struggling with. There are many different modalities of psychotherapy, and these often focus on different elements such as the root cause of mental ill health, as in relational Transactional Analysis (TA) for example, but others, such as many types of CBT, Person-Centred and Solution Focused psychotherapy, are not so focused on the cause. There continue to be differing thoughts and theories about what might be the optimal length of psychotherapeutic treatment (Howes, 2014; Leichsenring & Rabung, 2011). Traditionally, psychotherapy is often long term, lasting months, and even possibly years. Short-term work does exist, such as 6–12 sessions offered in employee assistance programmes (EAP), IAPT services and many charities for bereavement and mental well-being). Tensions and debate also continue to exist around the similarities and differences between psychotherapy and counselling, although this debate is not focused on here.

Relational psychotherapy is not new. Rather, it is a shift that has occurred in psychotherapy over the last 20 to 30 years. It has grown out of the need to offset goal-oriented therapy, offering a more eclectic, flexible approach, driven from the needs of the client, rather than the goal of the therapist. It understands that the therapist is not the expert, the client is. It also recognises that a therapist who looks objectively from a distance at a client's process may not engender the same change in one who seeks to be part of the process with the client. It is client-centred, ongoing, moment-by-moment attunement, where the therapist is a part of the process rather than separate from it. Its heart is the therapeutic alliance, and relational psychotherapy is hinged on the fact that it is the alliance between client and therapist, not the modality of therapy, that is the most important factor in treatment success.

The roots of relational therapy are integrative. It is a synthesis of British object relations theory, existential thinking, feminist and postmodern thinking, self-psychology and American interpersonal psychoanalytic thinking. The central tenet is the relationship between self and other, and in particular, therapist and client, healing through connection. Therapy focusses on this moment-by-moment relationship, using it as a way to unpick historical relationships. Any negative repetitive patterns from past relationships are played out in the therapy and can inform the present difficulties. If the client and therapist can gain understanding about what goes on between them, this may help them to understand what goes on outside the relationship. This enables the client to understand fundamental questions such as 'who am I' in relationship to others, 'what is my value to others and to myself' and 'what forms me'. Relationship to self and others, and patterns of relating are seen to be more powerful for change than insight alone. It also negates the belief that the power is within the individual and it is that person alone who needs fixing and who is responsible for their own happiness. Rather, it understands that our healthy, strong, stable connections with others, gives us power and agency. Our own thoughts, feelings, beliefs, self-states and energies are all interconnected with each other, and with those thoughts, feelings, beliefs, self-states and energies of others.

This fundamental shift in theory results from developments in science, neurobiology, and advances in knowledge of human development. There was also a growing understanding that clients were presenting with more complex presentations that theory could not explain nor treat. This relational movement was a move away from Freud, placing relationship at its heart.

Neuroscience is finally catching up with theory and is advancing at speed. We can now measure emotion scientifically, through levels of cortisol, epinephrine, and adrenaline. These have been identified as well as their receptors in the brain and body. Advances have also been made by Daniel Stern who began to map the interactions between mother and baby, helping developmental psychology to move forwards, and Allan Schore who has made it possible to understand the social and biological aspects of our emotional lives. We know that the infant's brain begins to form in utero and that fundamental parts of the pre-frontal cortex finish developing at around 2 years of age, although its complete development doesn't finish totally until our mid-20s. A lack of attachment, or indeed a traumatic attachment between caregiver and infant, during this period, can produce a gap in this development, causing fundamental life-long consequences in emotional regulation, capacity, compassion and empathy. This is because our cognition is built on our emotional intelligence, and our primitive gut responses. Mind and body work together, not separately. Our primitive gut responses are automatic fear responses which kick in when something unpleasant happens.

What actually is 'relational psychotherapy'?

Helena Hargaden and Joseph Schwartz identified key elements apparent in relational psychotherapy which have been usefully stated by Tudor (2014) in his commentary on the relational turn in psychoanalysis and psychotherapy which are:

- The centrality of the relationship
- Therapy as a two-way street involving a bi-directional process
- The vulnerability of both therapist and client are involved
- Countertransference is used not merely as information but in thoughtful disclosure and collaborative dialogue
- The co-construction and multiplicity of meaning

(Hargaden & Schwartz, 2007, p. 4)

When I speak of relational therapy in maternal mental illness, I am immediately thinking of using curiosity and creativity, working within the relationship between myself and my client, using attachment, bonding, and connection as well as working in the transferential domain. All of these elements together may help my client and me to unpick her relationship difficulties – with herself, with important others and with her baby. This may enhance a woman's ability to engage, attach and bond with herself, her baby and her wider family and friends.

Relational psychotherapy can be described as 'self-with-other'. What this actually means is that, in the here and now, we are relating together as therapist and client; we are experiencing our relationship; we are also hearing stories from the past, which are impacting us within our present moment relating. This is not about simply interpretation or illustration. This is about change being generated through the relational dyad, with a new form of relationship being generated through client and therapist interacting together, experiencing the impact they have on the other, and making meaning together about that impact and interaction. It is bidirectional, impacting both therapist and client, as active participants, and therefore both vulnerable to being shaped and changed by this process. We are actively co-creating new meaning, new stories and new interactions together. We are both impacted by the enactments that happen within our relationship. This type of therapy requires a commitment from the therapist, to be impacted by the client. It actively asks the therapist to work with their countertransference, to feel it, acknowledge, and sometimes disclose it in the service of the client. Also, the therapist needs to enter into the therapeutic relationship with absolutely no preconception of what is going to happen within that therapy. A truly relational psychotherapist has no agenda, other than facilitating the client to grow, in whatever way they want. This type of therapy also requires a commitment by the client to stay with the relationship, to know that dysfunctional relational patterns will be repeated over and over and within that process of repeating, something different may slowly emerge. Putting words and stories to the repeating patterns is a vital part of the emergence of something different and is a vital part of the healing process as is the depth of empathy. Therefore, it is really important that the therapist and client can account for the multiplicity of meaning that can be generated both individually and co-created together. For many with relational trauma, it is that the other did not stay, they walked away or abandoned the relationship that was so harmful. The fear is that people will then always walk away, always abandon, always neglect before any form of psychological repair can happen. Within psychotherapy, we call this process rupture and repair, and it is a fundamental part of the therapy. The ability to remain deeply empathic to the client's story, yet always retain a subjective sense of self.

Relational psychotherapy is not for everyone. Some therapists find it deeply disturbing working in the transferential domain and struggle to remain open to the vicissitudes of this type of work. It can feel messy and sticky, and at times the client may feel quite persecutory. For some therapists, using 'psychotechnologies' (Sanders, 2014) – such as manuals, instruments, protocols and obsessive measuring – can feel safe. Yet these can place a barrier between therapist and client, stopping the therapist being altered in any way shape or form by the client. Using psychotechnologies is not my type of psychotherapy, nor do I believe it is helpful for women with maternal mental illness, who are struggling with their distress. These women want to be heard, acknowledged, and witnessed in their distress. As well as changing from, and growing psychologically, in their reflective capacity. It is my deeply held belief that something transformational happens within relational psychotherapy, which does not necessarily happen in a one-person (Stark, 1999), more interpretive style of therapy, which we might call a more classical model.

A critique of relational psychotherapy

The relational style of psychotherapy has been critiqued by many (see Loewenthal & Samuels, 2014 for a full appraisal). Some believe it is no different from a more traditional style of psychoanalysis and assert that all therapeutic work is actually relational regardless of whether it is based on Freudian theory around the individual or Melanie Klein's view of the good and bad object. Zvi Carmeli and Rachel Blass assert that many of the ideas of traditional psychoanalysis are actually the same, but simply renamed:

> *Relational analysts will speak of organizing principles rather than representations or internal objects (Stolorow & Atwood, 1992 of unformulated experience rather than unconscious contents (Stern, 1997), of an interactive process of construction of a limited range of possible realities rather than the interpretation of psychic reality (Hoffman, 1991), but many of the same ideas are retained.*
>
> (2014, Chapter 10)

Others, such as Andrew Samuels (2014), believe that there is another part to relational, which he terms the 'shadow', which he feels may be harmful to clients. In his critique of relational psychoanalysis and psychotherapy, he discusses two elements that he finds problematic, which he says bring relational into a flatness, with 'no scratchy bits': (i) he sees a problem with focusing totally on the relationship as he believes this negates what he calls 'the phenomenon of solitude', of introversion; (ii) relational theory he believes has led therapists to hypocrisy, moralism and conformism due to their focus on providing a 'secure container' for the therapeutic relationship. He argues that there needs to be stress on the boundaries, as it is this element that produces a greater ability to become self-reflective and thus leads to growth within the client. He believes that the relational turn shows hypocrisy, in that relational therapists are unable to apply the same standards to themselves as to their clients, and are 'play-acting', particularly in respect of the topic of sex – the body and the behaviour. He also questions whether there is simply only 'one' relationship and believes that there are multiple relationships which are functioning simultaneously with each other (Clarkson, 1995). I would argue, in turn, that working relationally with my clients is often working at the boundaries which can be painful for both therapist and client and I would further argue, brings up all the 'scratchy bits' and much more. I would also argue that the phenomenon of solitude may not be what women need when they are struggling with this illness. One of the fundamental elements that is talked about by many women is their sense of isolation and aloneness in their illness. Working with other types of mental illness, I believe Samuels may indeed be correct. However, I would fundamentally disagree with this particular client group. I would agree with Samuels about his difficulty with the hypocrisy of some therapists in their inability or unwillingness to sit in the client's chair and experience what this is like. Here I do not mean a short-term relationship of therapy for the simple gathering of hours needed to become a therapist, a tick-box exercise that some students seem to believe is OK as part of their journey to become a psychotherapist. I am meaning a long-term, deep and often bumpy relationship in therapy with a professional who is focused on discovering all the multitude of rabbit roles and warrens within our psychological process.

Another critique is the use of the parental metaphor as analogous to that of the relationship between therapist and client (Parker, 2014). In psychotherapy, this is a useful concern, regarding power relations and the infantilisation of client. However, within maternal mental illness, I would argue that there is often this parallel process. The mother and child are often literally in the room with me, and I can see elements of our therapeutic relationship mirrored in her relationship with her infant. This, I would argue, is a useful part of the process, to see the relational dyad in front of me, and to be curious with the mother about her own relationship with her mother. I would argue that this is possibly one time when the use of the parental metaphor is useful rather than infantilising.

Del Loewenthal brings a critique to the relational through ethics and the ethics of practice (2014). Ethics is an area which is fundamental and complex in maternal mental illness and as such I have tried to address some of the ethical elements that I think about within my own practice with this client group (see Chapter 10 – ethical dilemmas in motherhood). This is an area which needs addressing and a fuller dialogue with practitioners working in this area may indeed expand and elucidate the complexities.

A clinical vignette

Lucy: Giving birth to twins in lockdown

Lucy came to therapy 2 months after the birth of her twins, who were born by Caesarean a few weeks early. Therapy was on zoom as we were still in the middle of the pandemic. Her husband had initially contacted me, as he was concerned that Lucy was not bonding with their babies, and he was fearful that her mental health was deteriorating. Another aspect was Lucy's quite serious lack of sleep. Lucy tried to sleep but found her mind racing in the small hours, consumed by anxiety that the moment she slept, she would be awakened again. Lack of sleep is normal, with small babies. However, exhaustion does not help a mother in her already difficult task of looking after a newborn, and lack of sleep and sleep disruption disrupt circadian rhythms, which may be a risk factor for women who are vulnerable to postpartum psychosis (Lewis, Foster & Jones, 2016). Luckily, Lucy had a doctor who understood this need for sleep and shortly after our work began gave her a short-term prescription of medication. This helped her and was the beginning of her pathway to feeling better, as she was able to connect better and engage more fully in our sessions.

Lucy had high levels of anxiety and stress and was not enjoying motherhood. She was finding having twins difficult and relied on her husband to help her with her daughters. One re-occurring theme was her anger about having twins. She said she never wanted two babies, and felt it was unfair. My first role was to help Lucy calm her distress down so that we could begin to work on the other difficulties she had, such as a reluctance to pick either of the babies up when they cried. She said her pregnancy had been difficult as she found out she was pregnant during the first pandemic lockdown, and nearly all her clinical appointments were on her own, with her husband waiting for her outside in the car park. She told me she was devastated when she found out they were having twins and during most of her pregnancy, she admitted to feeling a sense of foreboding.

I realised quickly that Lucy found it difficult to talk about her experiences of pregnancy and birth. She was distant and disconnected, her voice was monosyllabic, and monotone and I found it difficult to gain any connection with her at first. However, her presentation gave me really useful clues about her experience. She said she felt very scared, and out of control and was experiencing high levels of guilt about her difficulty with caring for her daughters. She told me she was not good at mothering, that it was not coming naturally, although she clearly felt that it should have been. I also noticed that, from the beginning, she talked about her babies in the plural, and rarely called them by their names. To me, this was a sign of her difficulty in bonding. It felt as though the girls were not Lucy's babies, and she described them almost as if they were someone else's, and a pair that she may have found difficult to separate.

The primary focus of our therapy together, once Lucy's distress lessened, was teaching Lucy to be in relationship with her babies. A part of Lucy's difficulty was her need to be perfect in everything she did. This need for perfection was a real block for her bonding with her babies, as every part of motherhood to her was mucky, sticky, smelly and my sense was that she found it a little boring and sordid. Lucy was a high-flying lawyer before she had the twins, and wanted to get back to work as quickly as was possible. Being a lawyer was a role where she was able to be perfect and she knew and understood her role very well. Motherhood was an altogether different and excruciating challenge for her. I felt the need to gently confront her perfectionism, which was almost to an obsessional level. I felt her need for perfection would be an unconscious wedge between her and the girls, as the babies could never live up to such high levels of perfectionism. My experience of

Lucy was of her trying to split away from her husband and daughters, using her work as an excuse to step back and instead let him step in to feed and raise the babies.

The babies were born early, and Lucy had struggled in hospital, feeling isolated and ashamed. She said she felt the staff in the maternity unit were judging her as being unable to care for the twins. I wondered if the staff were as bewildered as Lucy, struggling with the lack of information on how to keep themselves and their patients safe, with high levels of fear for everyone, staff, patients and partners alike. Lucy gave birth in the second lockdown in the UK.

Research shows that mums who went through pregnancy and labour during the pandemic had a difficult and anxious time with lack of choice in their options to give birth, with more interventions, such as caesareans recorded and difficulties in gaining pain control (Aydin et al., 2021). When the pandemic began, a great many hospitals in the UK, the USA and worldwide refused partners entry to antenatal appointments and the birth was often isolating, with all staff fully masked and robed up, with little human connection, and a lack of information about whether partners could attend or not. This caused significant stress and anxiety as well as a lack of certainty. Clearly, this had a profound effect on Lucy. My experience of her was that she was traumatised by her experience, seeming distant, struggling to connect, and with difficulty in narrating much to me. Her gaze was often away on something else, and Lucy seemed to find it difficult to keep any kind of eye contact. Hearing her talk about her experience, I realised Lucy had gone through the vast majority of her pregnancy and birth with extreme fear. Unfortunately, it was not until December 2020 that the NHS in the UK issued guidance saying that pregnant women should have one person with them during their hospital visits, by which time her twins had been born. Everything she and her husband had planned about their babies, the appointments, the labour and birth were all unhelpful, as Lucy had to do nearly all on her own. All the news items were about how many people were dying, and yet her husband was taking her to hospital to give birth. She said she was absolutely terrified she or the babies would get the virus in hospital and then die, but she had no choice, she had to have a caesarean.

Once Lucy began to bond with her babies she was able to separate them into individuals, with their own personalities. She lacked confidence in her mothering and easily handed either of the twins to her husband if she felt even slightly uncomfortable. She was unable to tolerate their crying and Lucy would become overwhelmed very quickly, particularly if the babies cried a lot. A turning point came, when she finally admitted to me that she was scared of her babies and felt unable to know what they wanted or needed from her. As time went on, she became very low, and cried a great deal in our sessions together. She kept saying she wanted to go back to before she was pregnant, to Lucy before the babies. Learning who she was as a mother and tolerating this was a large part of our therapy. She also needed to grieve the loss of her fantasy of pregnancy, birth and family. This wanting to go back to before is something I hear a lot from mums. They seem to convince themselves that life was perfect prior to birth. Yet often, it was not. Coming to terms with their new reality can take time, and for some, it can feel almost as if they are on a rollercoaster of emotions, and they just want to get off.

Another significant moment occurred when Lucy's lack of relationship with her own mother came sharply into focus. Lucy was convinced her mother was disinterested in her and with the twins. Lucy had isolated herself away from her parents, and rarely talked to her mother anymore. She talked about feeling angry, abandoned and neglected in favour of her older sister, who she described as her mother's favourite. Certainly, her descriptions of the family dynamics seemed to favour her older sister, and Lucy and her younger sister seemed to have bonded together in their feelings of abandonment. Again, I gently probed this dynamic of siblings and the mother's 'favourite'. I had a hunch that Lucy was passing something similar onto the younger of the twins, something from Lucy's own dynamic with her mother – second child that was abandoned and unloved due to being 'the difficult one', something we talk about in TA as transgenerational scripting. Certainly, it seemed that she was more tolerant of her older twin.

We explored how Lucy's dysfunctional relationship with her mother impacted on her own mothering. We also explored Lucy's lack of confidence and her anxiety. What transpired was that her own mother was also highly anxious and was unable to calm and regulate Lucy, leaving Lucy unable to regulate herself. Lucy's husband was the one she turned to for co-regulation, due to his absolute calmness and ability to remain calm in the face of difficulty. My role was also as co-regulator, particularly in the early sessions, when Lucy was on a level of hyper-alertness and seemed in turmoil. I found myself speaking very slowly and calmly with her, and my tone of voice and clarity of speech was gentle and soothing. Lucy would often start her sessions at a high pace, with a pressure of speech and a high-pitched voice. She was not experiencing postpartum mania, yet at times I wondered how close she may have been to becoming seriously unwell. Helping her to regulate her emotions, she said, allowed her to 'calm down, so everyone could calm down'. She meant the twins when she used the word 'everyone', and she began to notice how they responded to her when she was able to keep her anxiety in check.

It has not been easy going for Lucy. She often speaks about her anger at being the mother of twins, and frets about why it happened to her. She admitted to being jealous of those women 'lucky enough to have only one baby', and we spent time exploring all her different emotions, but particularly anger and sadness. During the writing of this book, our work has continued and has shifted onto Lucy's own birth story, which Lucy believes has a key role to play in her mental illness.

References

Aydin, E., Glasgow, K.A., Weiss, S.M., Khan, Z., Austin, T., Johnson, M.H., Barlow, J., and Lloyd-Fox, S. (2021). Giving birth in a pandemic: Women's birth experiences in England during COVID-19. *medRxiv*, https://doi.org/10.1101/2021.07.05.21260022

Battle, C.L., Salisbury, A.L., Schofield, C.A., and Ortiz-Hernandez, S. (2013). Perinatal antidepressant use: Understanding Women's preferences and concerns. *Journal of Psychiatric Practice*, 19(6), p. 443–453. https://doi.org/10.1097/01.pra.0000438183.74359.46

Carmeli, Z., and Blass, R. (2014). The relational turn in psychoanalysis: Revolution or regression? In Del Loewenthal, & Andrew Samuels (Eds), *Relational Psychotherapy, Psychoanalysis and Counselling: Appraisals and Reappraisals*. Hove, England: Routledge.

Clarkson, P. (1995). *The Therapeutic Relationship in Psychoanalysis, Counselling Psychology and Psychotherapy*. London: Whurr.

Department of Health (2013). IAPT Perinatal Positive Practice Guide. London. Retrieved from https://www.uea.ac.uk/documents/246046/11919343/perinatal-positive-practice-guide-2013.pdf/aa054d07-2e0d-4942-a21f-38fba2cbcceb

Dennis, C.-L., and Chung-Lee, L. (2006). Postpartum depression help-seeking barriers and maternal treatment preferences: A qualitative systematic review. *Birth*, 33, p. 323–331. https://doi.org/10.1111/j.1523-536X.2006.00130.x

Fowlie, H., and Sills, C. (2011). *Relational Transactional Analysis: Principles in Practice*. London: Karnac.

Goodman, J.H. (2009). Women's attitudes, preferences, and perceived barriers to treatment for perinatal depression. *Birth*, 36(1), p. 60–69. https://doi.org/10.1111/j.1523-536X.2008.00296.x

Hargaden, H., and Schwartz, J. (2007). Editorial. *European Journal of Psychotherapy and Counselling*, 9(1), p. 3–5. https://doi.org/10.1080/13642537.2010.518439

Hoffman, I.Z. (1991). Discussion: Toward a social-constructivist view of the psychoanalytic situation. *Psychoanalytic Dialogues*, 1, p.74–105. https://doi.org/10.1080/10481889109538886

Howes, R. (2014). How Long is Too Long in Psychotherapy. *Psychology Today*. Retrieved from https://www.psychologytoday.com/blog/in-therapy/201403/how-long-is-too-long-in-psychotherapy [accessed 06.02.18].

Kwan, B., Dimidjian, S., and Rizvi, S. (2010). Treatment preference, engagement and clinical improvement in pharmacotherapy versus psychotherapy for depression, *Behaviour Research and Therapy*, 48(8), p. 799–804. https://doi.org/10.1016/j.brat.2010.04.003

Leichsenring, F., and Rabung, S. (2011). Long-term psychodynamic psychotherapy in complex mental disorders: Update of a meta-analysis. *British Journal of Psychiatry*, 199(1), p. 15–22. https://doi.org/10.1192/bjp.bp.110.082776

Lewis, K.J.S., Foster, R.G., and Jones, I.R. (2016). Is sleep disruption a trigger for postpartum psychosis? *British Journal of Psychiatry*, 208(5), p. 409–411. https://doi:10.1192/bjp.bp.115.166314

Loewenthal, D. (2014). Relational ethics: From existentialism to post-existentialism. In D. Loewenthal & A. Samuels (Eds), *Relational Psychotherapy, Psychoanalysis and Counselling: Appraisals and Reappraisals*. Hove, England: Routledge.

Loewenthal, D., and Samuels, A. (2014). *Relational Psychotherapy, Psychoanalysis and Counselling: Appraisals and Reappraisal*. Hove, England: Routledge.

O'Mahen, H.A., and Flynn, H.A. (2008). Preferences and perceived barriers to treatment for depression during the perinatal period. *Journal of Women's Health*, 17(8), p. 1301–1309. https://doi.org/10.1089/jwh.2007.0631

O'Mahen, H.A., Grieve, H., Jones, J., McGinley, J., Woodford, J., and Wilkinson, E. (2015). Women's experiences of factors affecting treatment engagement and adherence in internet delivered behavioural activation for postnatal depression. *Internet Interventions*, 2(1), p. 84–90. https://doi.org/10.1016/j.invent.2014.11.003

Parker, I. (2014). It's the stupid relationship. In D. Loewenthal & A. Samuels (Eds), *Relational Psychotherapy, Psychoanalysis and Counselling: Appraisals and Reappraisals*. Hove, England: Routledge.

Pearlstein, T.N., Zlotnick, C., Battle, C.L., Stuart, S., O'Hara, M.W., Price, A.B., Grause, M.A., and Howard, M. (2006). Patient choice of treatment for postpartum depression: A pilot study. *Archive of Women's Mental Health*, 9, p. 303–308. https://doi.org/10.1007/s00737-006-0145-9

Ruiz, M. (1997). *The Four Agreements: A Practical Guide to Personal Freedom*. San Rafael, CA: Amber-Allen Publishing, Inc.

Samuels, A. (2014). Shadows of the therapy relationship. In D. Loewenthal and A. Samuels (Eds), *Relational Psychotherapy, Psychoanalysis and Counselling: Appraisals and Reappraisals*. Hove, England: Routledge.

Sanders, P. (2014). Ordinary stories of intermingling of worlds and doing what is right: A person-centred view. In D. Loewenthal & A. Samuels (Eds), *Relational Psychotherapy, Psychoanalysis and Counselling: Appraisals and Reappraisals*. Hove, England: Routledge.

Stark, M. (1999). *Modes of Therapeutic Action*. Northvale, NJ: Jason Aronson Inc.

Stern, D.B. (1997). *Unformulated Experience: From Dissociation to Imagination in Psychoanalysis*. Hillsdale, NJ and London: The Analytic Press.

Stolorow, R.D., and Atwood, G.E. (1992). *Contexts of Being: The Intersubjectivist Foundation of Psychological Life*. Hillsdale, NJ: The Analytic Press.

Tudor, K. (2014). A critical commentary on 'the relational turn'. In D. Loewenthal & A. Samuels (Eds), *Relational Psychotherapy, Psychoanalysis and Counselling: Appraisals and Reappraisals*. Hove, England: Routledge.

10 Ethical Dilemmas in Motherhood

If 'do no harm' is the guiding light in ethics in psychotherapy, what do we do when we are faced with a mother who is harming herself deliberately? How do we navigate through a difficult session when exploring when is enough in terms of IVF? How do we respond when all our buttons are pressed by our client, a teenager, who is suicidal because she is pregnant after being raped by her cousin, yet whose religious upbringing has placed shame on her and forbidden her to have an abortion? How do we navigate our own bias when a mother talks about having a baby she has no interest in because she is frightened her partner will leave her if she doesn't, or admits to becoming pregnant solely to try and keep a fractured, dysfunctional relationship due to a fear of abandonment?

Motherhood has always involved politics, power, oppression and marginalisation and is filled with unanswered questions, difficulties and dilemmas. In this chapter, I am going to look at some of the complexities a woman or couple faces, from pre-conception through to post-birth. I also want to invite therapists to think about the gritty and sometimes troublesome, knotty issues we can face, in the moment, and the tensions that might arise in us, using short case vignettes and by posing a few problematic questions. The purpose of this chapter is not to give answers. Instead, it is to promote thinking, exploration and dialogue about cultural, religious, familial and political belief systems. Are some of the issues prejudice? What exactly is my role? Am I doing my best and also doing no harm? The questions throughout are designed to focus our attention inwards, with emotional awareness (Cozolino, 2018), as part of an ongoing process to expose prejudice, bias and preference, much of which is unspoken or goes unnoticed.

Power and medicalisation

Everyone is vulnerable to power, to transgressions and to unconscious processes. What I am busy with is: am I able to remain open to curiosity and to be flexible enough to allow for continuous change in my own moral thinking and judgement? My clients will challenge me, this is inherent in the nature of my work. Holding a frame of mutuality with curiosity and openness to learning, in my mind, brings my client and me closer to equality in the balance of power and brings reflective and reflexive practice.

DOI: 10.4324/9781003154891-12

Ethical codes are the protective wrapper which make explicit the basic values and philosophical principles we believe in. These codes are normally predicated on specific deontological guidelines (guidelines for professional ethics) and their purpose is to guarantee human rights as well as to comply with the law of the country. These are useful as a foundation for ethics, although rigidity in their application can lead to abuse of power; they need to be fit for purpose. However, a question might be – do we need a specific code of ethics when working with motherhood? Is it any different from our other work with clients? Some may also believe that one of the difficulties with birth and motherhood is that it is over controlled already, particularly in the Western world and the over medicalisation of birth.

I am a feminist and believe that mental health and childbirth are both natural parts of life, and our experiences, both negative and positive, are a part of difference and diversity. Natality (Arendt, 1958) is the most important element of life – without which humans simply would not exist. However, for many centuries childbirth has been hijacked by a patriarchal medical system which continues to offer a discourse filled with increasing intervention and medicalisation. There has been an alarming rise in caesarean section (CS) rates worldwide (Sandall et al., 2018). In Egypt, the rate is now considered to be at 50%, and in Eastern Europe, the rates are also very high such as in Bulgaria (44.58%), Romania (44.5%) and Poland (38.92%) (Visser et al., 2018). The WHO estimates that around 15% of women need access to rapid intervention by medical services (AbouZahr, 1998). However, the increasing medicalisation now means that pregnancies that are straightforward are subject to routine interventions, with an increase in assisted delivery and surgery (Johanson, Newburn & Macfarlane, 2002).

Another difficulty a woman has is that the male body continues to be the norm in medical and scientific research, and the production of knowledge. This has meant that women's medical difficulties are missed, misdiagnosed or can remain completely unheard of, and unresearched, such as within childbirth. Throughout this book I have spoken about how deafening women's silence is, from pregnancy through to post birth in research. Gender bias and the medical model are a large part of this problem of silence, as it has led to women being pathologized, rather than normalised. Within the medical model, there is an expectation for women to change themselves, to accept their mental illness, rather than voice their concerns (Jackson, 2019). Voicing concerns leads to accusations of women being hysterical, and here we are back to the beginning of time (and Chapter 2) and the circularity of the male medical discourse on women and birth.

The rise in fertility treatment

Another element to acknowledge is that we now live in a fast-evolving world in fertility treatment. This has an impact on family systems and brings its own ethical challenges and changes which can be impactful to those who come from a cultural or societal background that is less progressive. The family now takes on many different forms. Thinking about sperm and egg donorship and surrogacy, for example, this change in fertility and family systems, and the development, particularly in some countries, whereby there is no longer anonymity of the donor, means that family systems are further challenged. Children will potentially be able to contact their donor, and the donor may well be able to contact their offspring, bringing unforeseen consequences to the wider family system. This causes tensions and can influence choice about where (what country) to conceive and how. These changes are happening swiftly and can seem heady and intense to a couple, particularly if they feel they are running out of time.

There is also now a trend to delay conception of the first child, which has consequences on fertility and, in particular, ART. Statistics from the OECD show that the simple mean average of women giving birth is now 30 or above and this trend is increasing, due to this postponement of conception. The OECD state that there has been a decline in fertility rates of the 20 to 29-year age group. Conversely, in the 30 to 39-year age group, these rates are slightly higher. In many countries (for example, Australia, Denmark, Finland, Germany, New Zealand, Norway and the UK), the fertility rates in 30–34 years olds are higher than in any other age group (OECD Family Database – SF2.3; 2022). In the UK, the statistics for women giving birth showed that the fertility rate for women over the age of 40 was the only age group where the rate increased (Office for National Statistics, 2020). However, women who give birth at 40 years and above seem to have more complications, more premature births, more interventions at birth and more congenital malformations (ESHRE Capri Workshop Group, 2005).

Although I have treated pre-conception and conception separately, there are many aspects which are similar for both, such as:

- The decision to have children, or not
- Natural conception or ART – IVF, surrogacy and genetics
- Issues for single-sex couples
- Cultural/religious issues
- Adoption

Pre-conception – complicated choices

Pre-conception is a time full of hope and possibility. Yet it is also a time of uncertainty. There is no guarantee that pregnancy will occur and as the statistics on miscarriage in Chapter 5 show, there is also no guarantee that the pregnancy will continue. Many of us will spend a great deal of time, thought and effort, throughout our lives, on not becoming pregnant. However, when the decision has been made to try for a baby, it can bring strong conflicting emotions. If there is a prior medical diagnosis, such as polycystic ovarian syndrome or endometriosis, for example, the woman is already likely to be experiencing anxiety around conception and what her diagnosis might mean.

One important feeling is ambivalence. Exploring this can be fruitful, confusing and fluctuating. Rozsika Parker has written an excellent book called 'Torn in Two – The Experience of Maternal Ambivalence' (1995/2005) which is a helpful resource with useful insights into ambivalence in motherhood. Working with a client with ambivalence can feel like being on an emotional rollercoaster, with indecisiveness and flux both valuable parts of the therapeutic process.

Clinical vignettes from pre-conception

Vignette 1

Luke and Sam wanted to explore Luke's desire for children and Sam's indecision, as this was causing tension between them and threatening their marriage. Luke felt that time was running out. He wanted to have children when they both still had time and energy, and not leave it too late, when their life might be so fixed that it would never happen. Sam really was unsure whether or not he actually wanted children. Sam was able to admit his ambivalence about parenthood and it transpired that Sam was afraid to talk about this with Luke for fear of being judged abnormal or strange.

Luke's family was close and family-oriented, as well as open in their thinking about single-sex couples having children. However, Sam's family was horrified about the idea and put a great deal of pressure on Sam to think carefully about this decision. Sam was also struggling with the ideas of conception and surrogacy. He talked about feeling caught up with all the decisions they had to make, whose sperm to use, or whether to go with a donor sperm. He was suffused with fear that he would not bond with the child and wanted to explore whether this was even possible and whether he would begin to resent Luke or the infant, due to the impact on them as a couple. Sam was caught in passivity. He never doubted that Luke would be a great dad. His ambivalence was around doubt in himself.

Vignette 2

David's family continued to make jokes about their childlessness, without ever thinking to ask David or his wife Cheryl about their desire for a family. This left both Cheryl and David feeling inadequate, because they had been struggling with infertility for years and had been through expensive rounds of IVF. David's family had a complete lack of boundaries and continued to cross David and Cheryl's private, intimate and deeply personal boundaries. In fact, Cheryl and David's lack of children had become a hot topic for family conversation, with Cheryl and David totally excluded from the discussion. Many couples I speak to talk of never being asked about their choices by family members. Rather, assumptions are made, with no real knowledge, which many couples can find difficult and sometimes hurtful.

Vignette 3

It is often assumed that everyone wants to be a parent, yet of course, this is not true at all. However, in many families, parenthood is not talked about openly, and may be a taboo subject. Clara told me she thought about just doing it anyway, giving into her husband and his family in the hope that her feelings towards the child might grow, once the baby was born. I struggled with this, as a mother of three and knowing how hard motherhood was. My thoughts were with the unborn child, wondering what the impact of Clara's ambivalence might mean long term for her child's own sense of self.

Parent ambivalence is more spoken about now, although it is still cloaked with shame and guilt. Stereotypical views continue about women and men who do not want children, as if that is abnormal. Also, many people assume they are the only one who feels this way and can torture themselves, continually asking why they might feel like this? The woman will often continue to struggle with her decision-making process and may well continue to grieve her decision.

Questions for therapists to reflect on with clients:

How often do we think clearly about who we are as a person, and who we might be as a parent?

What are our thoughts towards becoming a parent?

Should we have children, or should we not?

Is there something wrong with me if I don't want children?

What will happen to me in old age if I don't have a child to support me?

How can I come to terms with never giving birth, would I regret this later?

How can I come to terms with the knowledge that I will never hold or love a child of my own and will never receive that unconditional love of a child in return?

Conception

Conception is a time suffused with different extremes of emotion, such as excitement to finally be pregnant, but fear about what this may mean. As with many other emotions in motherhood, these two conflicting emotions can run together throughout pregnancy and longer. This is also a time of immense choice. Ambivalence will often continue, and it may feel harder to choose, with the greater freedom there is with career choices and flexibility. Young adults today are particularly concerned about global warming and the future of the environment and some are thinking much more carefully about whether they want to bring a child into a world already so full of people. The COVID-19 pandemic has also highlighted fears about the future. Although some they will feel as if there has been no choice about conception.

Specific challenges for the parent(s)

A single person thinking about the possibility of having a baby:

- Who will be involved in their decision and in the process of becoming pregnant?
- Some may have little or no intention of involving another
- There may be no way of involving the father: he may be unknown, or possibly a stranger. She may have been raped or sexually abused
- Choices between natural conception: conceiving with a friend or colleague. Again, this can be fraught with choices and difficulty around the insemination process. There are some tough decisions to be made. If they wish to involve a friend, they will be involved and committed with each other and the child for possibly many years to come, with all the pressure that may place on the friendship
- Choices about IVF: where to go, how much to pay, who to trust, how many rounds to undergo

A single-sex couple:

- How to conceive: ART, donation or surrogacy?
- For single-sex male couples: whose sperm to use. Do we use one person's, or do we opt for using neither and choose donation, for equitability
- For single-sex female couples: whose egg to use; perhaps use one woman's egg and then transplant into the other. Where to find the sperm donor: ask someone known, how might that be? How to navigate that relationship in the future?
- Does the donor want/expect to be part of the baby's life, offering financial and time commitments?
- When to explain the baby's heritage and how to navigate their right to contact/not contact the donor(s)?

Dilemmas with ART

Questions the woman/couple may be exploring

- The tension between human rights to reproduce and the best interests of eventual children – possibility of discrimination
- How many IVF cycles to complete?
- How many eggs to fertilise?
- What happens to the unused fertilised eggs – destroy them or offer to other infertile couples?
- Implications of cost (financial as well as emotional and physical) and access to services
- Do I get to choose the person: issues of suitability; possible genetic abnormalities; use of illicit substances by the donor

- Rights of the donor/surrogate towards my child
- My child's right to accessing information about the donor
- The implications of hormone and drug therapy and the effects, both emotionally and physically, on the woman and the impact this may have on the couple's relationship

These processes are not straightforward. If a couple wants to use a donor, some countries insist on open donorship with all that this entails. This might have implications on where the couple chooses to go to have IVF. It has implications for the family long term because the child is then able to seek out their donor at a later date. Those wishing to use surrogacy also need to know it is not legal everywhere. For example, at the time of writing, Pakistan, Turkey, Saudi Arabia, Sweden, Austria and France are against surrogacy.

Questions for therapists to reflect on:

How do we put our own bias aside when a client who is morbidly obese, and so determined to have a child, continues to pay for round after round of IVF treatment in a private fertility clinic to no avail?

What if the woman is pregnant and having intense doubts about being pregnant?

What do we do when a client is harming themselves, yet is unable to see the self-harm, because their vision is so clouded?

At what point do we help the client to grieve and to tolerate their infertility?

Is it our role to help them to understand that it is futile to continue to hope?

Clinical vignettes from conception

Vignette 1

Clare and John came together to explore their infertility and the strain it was putting on their relationship. Clare wanted to continue with another round of IVF, but John was unable to contemplate this as he felt it was destroying them as a couple. Conception for them was proving to be bumpy and tough. John wanted Clare to be able to come to a decision to stop. Helping a couple to come to this choice can be difficult. Luckily Clare and John had a strong bond, but John was becoming concerned that Clare was fixated on pregnancy to the detriment of all else. Clare continued to hold hope. John did not. Clare's hope was beginning to make her unwell. Fertility difficulties cause mental health issues such as anxiety, with a need to hurry up, due to a sense of age and losing time. This was Clare's difficulty. She was nearly 45 and had been through many rounds of IVF already. Fear is often present: of being good enough; of what will happen; of the toll on the relationship. John was scared that this was never going to end, and that the clinics would never say no to another round due to commercialism, and he felt this was unfair on Clare and was stoking her hope.

Both parties may already have mental health difficulties. This adds further complexities, particularly if one party is on medication that may be risky to the fetus. Questions arise of what that might mean for their fertility: what impact it might have on the fetus; how will they know the impact; what if they would need to come off medication for conception to occur; how long might that take; what are the risks that might be involved with this. There are so many nuances to conception that often do not surface until a couple has already started their journey.

Other aspects

If there is a genetic risk within the family, this can place a huge strain on both the couple and family, particularly if it uncovers previously unknown heritability of specific genetic traits that impact the fetus/infant. What might this mean to the wider family? How might this affect choices? There may be a fear around disability and how the couple might cope.

There can also be difficulties around food, alcohol, smoking, and health. These may challenge the therapist's own bias or moral values. Most adults know and understand that drinking alcohol can cause deformities in the fetus (see Chapter 4 regarding FAS) and that smoking is harmful. However, what if our client refuses to stop either. Food, smoking and alcohol are also areas of possible shame and can be anxiety provoking due to lack of information or misinformation on social media sites. Although these issues may be more heightened within pregnancy, the anxiety can often begin at conception. Is it our place as psychotherapists to educate or even step in?

Pregnancy – Transition

In pregnancy, the questions and difficulties alter again and split into the fetus and the mother. Some are separate, some affect both. In the UK, at the time of writing, a fetus does not have a legal personality separate from its mother, until it is born. Women are free to make choices about the fetus, which may be against medical advice, so long as they are able to show an informed decision. However, in 2017 there were 125 countries in the world in which abortion was prohibited and 42% of women of reproductive age lived in those countries (Singh et al., 2018). Some babies are conceived through rape or sexual abuse: the mother may choose to keep the baby or have no alternative due to a prohibition on termination. Each country will have a differing legal standpoint. Another area of challenge is the point in time in which a fetus becomes 'a person' in law with legal rights. Again, each country will have a different view and it is important to know this, particularly if we are working with people who are based in different countries, in this advent of psychotherapy on zoom.

Questions for therapists to reflect on:

Whose choice is it to terminate?

What if the pregnancy was a mistake: a one-night stand, perhaps?

What if the pregnancy was from rape or sexual abuse?

What if the woman knows the abuser or he is a relation or family friend?

What about if the woman does not want to involve the father?

What about religious or cultural implications and dilemmas if termination is forbidden no matter what?

How do we support women who are so deeply shamed about their weight gain in pregnancy?

As an example, recently in Northern Ireland, there was a great deal of debate around termination, due to the legal ban on all abortions. Even with abnormalities that meant the fetus would probably not survive to a point where it would be possible for it to live outside the womb, abortions were illegal. Women were also required to continue to carry a baby if the medical profession knew that baby would be born in severe pain and would almost certainly not survive the birth process or would die shortly after birth, due to genetic abnormalities. This only changed when the power-sharing government collapsed, and the UK government stepped into the power vacuum and changed the law, so it was in line with the rest of the UK. However, although the law has changed, the Northern Ireland government still has not put funding in place to provide the services required. At least it is now no longer possible for a mother to be prosecuted for acquiring the morning after pill, whereas prior to the change in law, it was illegal.

Similarly, in September 2021, a bill was passed in Texas in the United States, banning all terminations after week six of a pregnancy, even if the pregnancy was due to rape or incest. The focus of this law is on the ability to sue a doctor who performs a termination, rather than suing the woman who receives the procedure. The difficulty is that many women do not even know they are pregnant at 6 weeks, and at this stage, the fetus still has no heartbeat as such. This overturned the law made in the US by the Supreme Court in 1973, when all women had the right to an abortion up to 22 weeks of gestation.

Other aspects

Things to consider are miscarriage, and stillbirth. How is the mother supported through this within the healthcare system and in therapy in her country? Some women, after a miscarriage, talk about feeling discounted by the health service, being given little or no information about why they miscarried or feeling violated due to the obstetric procedures that they have had to endure. Although extremely uncommon, women carrying twins who lose one baby late in pregnancy may need to continue carrying the deceased baby and give birth to that baby at the same time as the surviving twin, which is understandably extremely traumatising.

Women who smoke in pregnancy are often judged and perceived to be deliberately harming their babies. In pregnancy, a mother can feel deeply shamed by those, including medical professionals, who seem to have little in the way of a filter system for comments. This might be around behaviours that are perceived to be not in the interest of the unborn child. One area of shame I consistently see is around weight gain during pregnancy, particularly if the woman believes that what is actually happening may be due to gestational diabetes, or if the woman has had a previous diagnosis of gestational diabetes. Weight is such a sensitive subject, and although it is important that women do not become obese in pregnancy, women can feel judged negatively, or viewed as not ok. For some, this can lead to obsession about weight gain, which can be transferred onto the infant once born.

Finally, there is also the aspect of epigenetics which begin with the environment during pregnancy, and continue throughout life, shaping our genes, and can have far-reaching consequences for the growing fetus, through inheritance and development.

Birth

Who holds the power and the choice within the birth process? Women would like to think they hold both. However, this is not the experience for all. In Chapter 5, I explored maternal trauma, and in particular, birth trauma. I spoke about how many women believe that their health practitioner played a fundamental role in their birth trauma. In the Western world, most babies are delivered in hospital. There is an explicit expectation about this, and mothers often say they had little or no opportunity to make a choice between home and hospital birth, as the choice was not theirs to make. In a recent study on midwifery in the UK, midwives spoke of feeling constrained by a lack of capacity and excessive demands on their time, coping with an approach suitable for business, influenced by throughput and the formulaic discourse of self-protection, rather than prioritising the safety of mothers and babies (Shallow, Deery & Kirkham, 2018). Research from the World Health Organization found that there was a drive in many countries to concentrate maternity services into larger, more medicalised multidisciplinary units, which has resulted in homebirth services being almost eliminated (Phelan & O'Connell, 2015).

When women discover this lack of choice, it often causes frustration and anger, as their birth experience bears no resemblance to their expectations. In order to facilitate more patient choice – birth plans have been in use in various Western countries since the 1980s. These are useful for a woman to express her aspirations for birth and facilitate communication with healthcare practitioners during the birthing process. Yet, many women talk about hearing little or no mention of their plan during the birth process and speak of feeling out of control and unable to voice how they want the process to go. This gives them the sense of being 'done to'.

Questions for therapists to reflect on:

How do I help a woman who is blaming her baby for her birth trauma?

How do I feel about a woman giving birth to a baby and giving it up for adoption?

What about working with a woman in Brazil or Romania where there are very high levels of C-section, who wants to have a vaginal delivery but whose doctor was helping her to 'choose' a Caesarean?

How do I support a woman who has experienced medical negligence yet believes she is the one who was at fault?

Post birth

There are many questions which may arise post birth, many of which have already been addressed to some extent within the rest of this book. Some other aspects which can bring gritty experiences and difficulties are:

- Bringing up children
- Parental role biases
- The involvement of family, and/or community with raising the children
- Parental roles in medical decision-making
- Parental rights and decisions regarding any kind of medical input
- Unwanted children – adoption and fostering.
- Moral differences in couples
- Expectation of religious practices (circumcision, for example) or
- Differences in gender status
- Economic anxiety: how can I/we afford the cost to bring up a child

There are also many other aspects that the couple might decide to explore, such as identity and how this will change with parenthood and what this might mean for them as an individual and as a couple.

Conclusion

This chapter is purposefully open to interpretation. There are no right or wrong answers to many of the questions I pose. Rather, there is opportunity for dialogue and consideration about some of the questions that may get raised in therapy. It is a chance for therapists to explore and learn about their prejudices, biases, strengths and weaknesses as part of their ongoing process of self-reflection and awareness.

References

AbouZahr, C. (1998). Maternal mortality overview. In C.J.L. Murray & A. Lopez (Eds), *Health Dimensions of Sex and Reproduction: The Global Burden of Sexually Transmitted Diseases, HIV, Maternal Conditions, Perinatal Disorders, and Congenital Anomalies*. Cambridge, MA: Harvard School of Public Health. (Global burden of disease and injury series. Vol 3.)

Arendt, H. (1958). *The Human Condition*. Chicago: University of Chicago Press.

Cozolino, L. (2018). Creativity in the training of psychotherapists. In Terry Marks-Tarlow, Marion Solomon, and Daniel J. Siegel, (Eds), *Play & Creativity in Psychotherapy*. New York: W.W. Norton & Company.

ESHRE Capri Workshop Group. (May/June 2005). Fertility and ageing. *Human Reproduction Update*, 11(3), p. 261–276. https://doi.org/10.1093/humupd/dmi006

Jackson, G. (2019). The female problem: How male bias in medical trials ruined women's health. *The Guardian*. Retrieved from https://www.theguardian.com/lifeandstyle/2019/nov/13/the-female-problem-male-bias-in-medical-trials [accessed 16.12.21].

Johanson, R., Newburn, M., and Macfarlane, A. (2002). Has the medicalisation of child-birth gone too far? *BMJ (Clinical Research Ed.)*, 324(7342), p. 892–895. https://doi.org/10.1136/bmj.324.7342.892

OECD Family Database – SF2.3: Age of mothers at childbirth and age-specific fertility. *OCED.Stat*. Retrieved from https://www.oecd.org/els/family/database.htm [accessed 2021].

Office for National Statistics. (2020). Births in England and Wales: 2019. Retrieved from https://www.ons.gov.uk/peoplepopulationandcommunity/birthsdeathsandmarriages/livebirths/bulletins/birthsummarytablesenglandandwales/2019 [accessed 07.12.21].

Parker, R. (1995/2005). *Torn in Two – The Experience of Maternal Ambivalence*. London: Virago Press.

Phelan, A., and O'Connell, R. (2015). Childbirth: Myths and Medicalization. WHO/Europe, No. 81 https://www.euro.who.int/__data/assets/pdf_file/0007/277738/Childbirth_myths-and-medicalization.pdf

Sandall, J., Tribe, R.M., Avery, L., Mola, G., Visser, G.H., Homer, C.S., Gibbons, D., Kelly, N.M., Kennedy, H.P., Kidanto, H., Taylor, P., and Temmerman, M. (2018). Short-term and long-term effects of caesarean section on the health of women and children. *Lancet*, Oct 13, 392(10155), p. 1349–1357. https://doi.org.10.1016/S0140-6736(18)31930-5. PMID: 30322585.

Shallow, H., Deery, R., and Kirkham, M. (2018). Exploring midwives' interactions with mothers when labour begins: A study using participatory action research. *Midwifery*, 58, p. 64–70. https://doi.org/10.1016/j.midw.2017.10.017

Singh, S., Remez, L., Sedgh, G., Kwok, L., and Onda, T. (2018). Abortion Worldwide 2017 – Uneven Progress and Unequal Access. Published by Guttmacher Institute. https://www.guttmacher.org/sites/default/files/report_pdf/abortion-worldwide-2017.pdf

Visser, G.H.A., Ayres-de-Campos, D., Barnea, E.R., de Bernis, L., Di Renzo, G.C., Vidarte, M.F.E., Lloyd, I., Nassar, A.H., Nicholson, W., Shah, P.K., Stones, W., Sun, L., Theron, G.B., and Walani, S. (2018). FIGO position paper: How to stop the caesarean section epidemic. *Lancet*, Oct 13, 392(10155), 1286–1287. https://doi.org/10.1016/S0140-6736(18)32113-5. PMID: 30322563.

11 Treating the Cause of Maternal Mental Illness

I use 'treating the cause' to mean focussing on the source of mental illness rather than offering only symptomatic relief. Why? Clients often come with an expectation that we will do something for them, take their symptoms away and make them feel better. However, it is important to do a great deal more than this. Symptomatic relief is short-term relief. It does not last long, and it does not look for the root cause of the problem. Addressing the cause allows a woman the possibility to conceive a future with reduced mental illness, even possibly no mental illness at all and is fundamental to my way of working.

In mental illness, research shows that medical practitioners seem to follow only symptoms when making decisions about treatment (Waszczuk et al., 2017). Although obviously not a mental disorder, I would like to use a headache as an example of what I mean. If I have a headache, I might choose to take off-the-shelf medication to alleviate the pain (treating the symptom). However, if I continue to have the same headache for weeks or months, I might eventually go to the doctor and expect to be sent for tests to discover why I have the headache (the cause).

If I go to a doctor with symptoms of mental illness, the doctor will use the medical model to treat my symptoms, and I am likely to get a prescription for psychiatric medication, an antidepressant for example, a drug that will affect my brain and body. Yet, what do we actually know about the toxicity of psychiatric drugs, or if they do more harm than good (Moncrieff, 2009/2020). The difficulty with mental illness is that the medical model may not be fit for purpose (Caplan, 2019; Timimi, 2020). Many doctors and psychiatrists follow the medical model – that it is a deficit or a biological cause that underlies all mental health conditions. The psychiatric medication they give supposedly addresses the 'chemical imbalance' in the brain. However, what scientific evidence is this based on, and does such medication actually address the cause? Moncrieff highlights the lack of evidence, saying, '*Despite popular beliefs and the claims made by pharmaceutical companies and professional organisations, there is little evidence, therefore, to support even the most well-accepted biochemical theories about the origins of psychiatric symptoms. They remain theories or hypotheses, rather than fact*' (2009/2020, p. 23).

DOI: 10.4324/9781003154891-13

This theory of a chemical imbalance persists even though there is no evidence to prove it (Davies, 2013; Kirsch, 2010), and it is even called a 'myth' (Carlat, 2010). Let's go back to that headache – if we do not address the cause of the headache, the pain medication we take may not be adequate. We may even need to take the pain medication for the rest of our lives in order to keep the headache at bay, and after a certain amount of time, we also may need to increase the headache medication, as our bodies will get used to it and more will be required to gain the same effect.

Instead, let us take a different biopsychosocial view about mental illness: that such illnesses are part of human diversity. That mental ill health is the normal consequence of the difficult and, at times, tragic personal and social events in our lives, or indeed a suitable response to traumatic events. Then, rather than treating the symptoms of this, as symptoms would also, therefore, be viewed as normal, it might be more helpful to look back into the woman's history to find out if there are clues about why she is feeling the way she does. These clues offer choices and can help her navigate a pathway through her challenging experiences.

Let us take anxiety, for example. So many of my clients come in telling me they are anxious and some even shake bodily in front of me. These women seem to think they were born with anxiety or at least that they have 'always' been anxious. However, anxiety is a symptom, just like many other mental health disorders – depression, addiction, and stress are good examples. There will be an underlying cause for the anxiety, and we need to know what it is and focus on the cause. Anxiety is fear. We need to ask what our clients are afraid of, so we can help them learn to firstly regulate themselves, then to explore with them if they can address whatever it is that they are so afraid of. Sometimes clients are taught to be afraid by their parents. Yet, the fear is not theirs and they might no longer need to be fearful. If we track back to the cause of a client's feelings, often that can unlock the present moment for them. It can bring understanding, and it can bring connection. Once we have connection, the intolerable can seem far less intolerable.

Firstly, I would like to highlight some of the research into a woman's history of mental illness and its role in pregnancy and the postnatal period. I then want to give a client example of how unlocking the cause of illness allowed the woman to move forwards with her life and to stop experiencing her maternal mental illness. The chapter finishes with a brief conclusion.

Research into prior mental illness

Research shows us that women with mental illness during pregnancy and the postnatal period will have often experienced a history of mental illness. In fact, this past history of mental illness is one of the strongest predictors of maternal mental illness (Chojenta et al., 2019; Cohen et al., 2006; Di Florio et al., 2013). Therefore, part of the cause of maternal mental illness may be historical illness, past trauma, or difficult childhood experiences growing up, all of which may be re-manifesting in some way in the perinatal period. If we think about those historical illnesses or past traumas, they are almost always due to dysfunctions in relationships. Difficult childhood experiences would include those children who have had emotional, physical and sexual abuse within their childhoods. I would also include those children who, at first glance, may seem to have had a good childhood. Nonetheless, they are deeply anxious and distressed due to their sense of not being OK, feeling in a one-down position, or feeling abandonment and neglect. Parents often do their utmost to raise their children well. However, time commitments, both parents working full time, and all the other pressures of life in the 21st century can mean that, even though those parents never mean to negatively impact their children's lives, they often do. Then add in the often multiple confounding factors, such as lack of sleep, medical difficulties in pregnancy, anxiety around the birth, addiction and/or relational difficulties and sometimes intimate partner violence, as well as fear of not bonding with the infant, breastfeeding difficulties and a sense of responsibility and overwhelm, plus the expectation that most women will take on the primary responsibility for looking after the children, it is unsurprising that many women feel overwhelmed and distressed.

Some research suggests that the changes in hormones can be enough to trigger dysregulation (Bloch et al., 2000; Schiller, Meltzer-Brody & Rubinow, 2015). Schiller et al. also hypothesise that some women are more sensitive to certain hormones and suggest the identification of what they call a postpartum depression phenotype, which they distinguish from other type of postpartum depression (2015). However, there is a surprising lack of research into the fluctuations of hormones in the perinatal period, and it would seem that medical research does not really understand all the impacts of these fluctuations. It is quite possible that a history of mental illness and hormones work together in some way, with other factors such as exhaustion and lack of sleep.

It is not only women with historical mental health difficulties that are more likely to experience perinatal mental health conditions. Women with chronic physical conditions are also more likely to be diagnosed with perinatal mental illness (20.4% of those diagnosed with such a condition) (Brown et al., 2019). Women may come into psychotherapy with depression or anxiety and with fibromyalgia after trauma during pregnancy or birth (Al-Allaf et al., 2002), for example. It is known that fibromyalgia may be triggered by high levels of stress in both its physical and emotional form, so it may well be that an experience of birth trauma was part of the cause of the fibromyalgia (Furness et al., 2018). There is a high co-morbidity of fibromyalgia and psychiatric illness (Galvez-Sánchez, Duschek & Reyes Del Paso, 2019).

Women with a history of severe mental health conditions prior to pregnancy are at risk of relapse during pregnancy and postnatally. A cohort of women with a history of major depression found that 43% had a relapse during pregnancy (Cohen et al., 2006). Women with a history of bipolar disorder were at an even greater risk with 50% at risk of relapse (Di Florio et al., 2013). Twenty percent of women with a pre-existing bipolar disorder experience a severe postnatal mental illness (psychosis, mania or hospitalisation) (Wesseloo et al., 2016). For women who have experienced schizophrenia, the risk postpartum for psychotic relapse is particularly high (Matevosyan, 2011). There are also other types of mental disorders that risk relapses such as prior eating disorders, obsessive compulsive disorders and anxiety. No matter what the mental disorder was prior to pregnancy, there seems to be a risk for a relapse, and so it would seem pertinent to address these difficulties as part of the psychotherapeutic process if the woman is in agreement.

What is clear from the research noted above is that it is important for us to enquire about any historical mental illness which may have a bearing or have similarities to the woman's experience of maternal mental illness. However, this is not the only important factor to consider. Knowing how a woman experienced her childhood and any influencing factors such as transgenerational history of maternal mental illness can also be useful in formulating a suitable pathway for treatment within psychotherapy. If a woman has experienced past trauma, it is quite possible that her experience in pregnancy and postnatally may also be traumatic. Addressing the original trauma may positively impact her maternal experience.

My own research on maternal mental illness included narratives of women's experiences (Haynes, 2019). All of the women in my research reported having historical mental illness of varying sorts. Exploring and addressing the cause of their illness was stated as a helpful factor in treatment. Several of the participants also reported that treatment using symptomatic relief, such as medication, was not enough to help them.

Enquiries into historical causes

Many women do not recognise their past difficulties within the perinatal period. For instance, a woman I saw with extreme health anxiety within pregnancy seemed unable to realise the importance of her historical struggles with ongoing asthma and a sense that she was 'sickly' in childhood. When we began exploring her childhood, there were multiple instances when she related feeling as if she would die due to differing ailments, particularly asthma. Health anxiety is a common feature of pregnancy, particularly with the woman fearing that she or her baby might die in childbirth or that she or the baby would be diagnosed with a terminal illness detected during an ultrasound appointment. Reassurance is often sought by pregnant or new mothers online, particularly during COVID-19, when women had little access to medical care. And this online seeking for information may exacerbate a woman's feelings around health anxiety, as the information is not always accurate or helpful and can increase anxiety rather than offer the reassurance needed.

The following clinical vignette tells a story I have now heard multiple times, in many similar guises.

Client vignette

Pippa – 'Abandoned'

Pippa came to me early on in her pregnancy with quite serious catastrophic thoughts about death and extreme levels of anxiety. In her first appointment, she sat on the edge of her seat and literally shook with fear and apprehension.

At first glance, I could have mistakenly assumed that Pippa had everything she could possibly want. She spoke of a privileged background as an only child and said she was lucky enough to go to a really good school. She had no idea why she catastrophised to such an extent, and in particular, she could not tell me why she was convinced either her baby or she would die. Death, her fear of it and her prevailing sense that it was imminent was the first part of our therapeutic exploration together.

In our second session, Pippa told me she was sent to boarding school at 7 years old because her father had been posted to China, and her mother chose to go with him. Pippa told me her parents were concerned Pippa would get behind at school if she came with them to China. Instead, her parents organised for her to go to a local girls' school that offered boarding for those children whose parents lived away. Pippa was very matter of fact about relating her experience of boarding and told me that she had known absolutely nothing about going to the school until she arrived there one day with her parents in the car. It was not until she sat down for tea with the other children that she realised her parents were no longer around. She said that she became quite frantic, asking where her parents had gone, but although the staff members were kind and tried to soothe her, she said she was inconsolable. She also told me that she had thought her parents would be back for her the next day, and it only dawned on her that she would be staying a great deal longer the next day. As was common at the time in many boarding schools, she had absolutely no contact with her parents for the first 3 weeks of school.

I knew when she told me this that Pippa may have been psychologically traumatised by her experience of being left alone at school, at such a young age, with no knowledge of when her parents would be back for her. My hypothesis, early on, was that Pippa's catastrophising was caused by her early trauma, although this was supposition and interpretation on my part at this point. I wondered with her what this had felt like at 7 years of age. She told me it was hell on earth. Yet, when I asked Pippa whether there was any link between this and her sense of intense apprehension, she totally denied it. In fact, she was so determined to prove me wrong that she spent several months painting a picture of a wonderful childhood with the best parents ever.

To some extent, she may have experienced elements of her childhood as wonderful. However, I had the distinct impression that I had the 7-year-old girl in front of me who was terrified to say anything against her parents in case she was abandoned forever by them. Pippa had an intense need to keep them in the position of good objects.

It was not until we began to talk about her experiences of boarding school that her conviction about her childhood began to slip. A turning point in our therapy was when I asked her what her thoughts were about schooling her soon-to-be-born infant. She told me very quickly that she and her husband were sending their child to the local school. She then said she would never inflict boarding school on one of her children.

The second turning point occurred when we began to explore Pippa's catastrophising and her sense of impending doom. She said her catastrophising felt like 'death', or at least hell. I gently wondered with her whether those first 3 weeks at boarding school, which she had described months before as 'like hell' for her may have been the precipitating factor in her catastrophising. She broke down and wept and told me that it was not only the first 3 weeks that were hell. She admitted that she continued to cry herself to sleep every night at school, convinced that she had done something seriously wrong, or been so incredibly naughty that she had been punished by being abandoned at boarding school. She said every night she tried to work out what she had done and why she had been punished so severely. It took her quite a while to begin to accept that she was not to blame.

The more we continued to explore her catastrophising, the more she saw similarities in her childhood feelings, which she had mostly buried, and how she felt now, terrified that she was going to die or that her baby would die. Pippa had also assumed her anxiety was simply normal and part of who she was as she had always been highly anxious. In fact, she talked about how her parents made fun of her anxiety and even she called herself needy. My role was to help her understand that her anxiety was caused by her traumatic experiences and that it was an understandable response to her trauma. This did not make her born anxious. Instead, her anxiety stemmed from her experience of boarding school at such a young age.

Some children flourish at boarding school. Others find it a traumatic and disturbing experience and are haunted by it, speaking about feeling isolation, loneliness, abandonment and fear. Age of first attendance is a factor. Those sent very early, at six or seven may feel particularly traumatised and abandoned by their parents. They may ask themselves what they did wrong to warrant their parents sending them away (Schaverien, 2015).

The consequence of her experience was that Pippa struggled being on her own, even though she was a grown woman with a partner and baby. She described herself as quite 'clingy'. Yet, I could understand why she might have felt the need to cling if she was never quite sure when her parents would vanish again.

Conclusion

Discovering why clients are unwell is almost like being a detective working on a complicated case. I want to track right back to the earliest parts of life and the relational transferential dynamics of the client's family, to unlock and unpick what happened to her and why she might be struggling now with her infant because, as Irigaray so rightly says, '*If we go on speaking the same language together we are going to reproduce the same history*' (1985, p. 205). Once we uncover the cause, we can begin to formulate a treatment direction which I go onto show in Chapter 13 – the therapeutic role.

References

Al-Allaf, A.W., Dunbar, K.L., Sallum, N.S., Nosratzadeh, B., Templeton, K.D., and Pullar, T. (2002). A case-control study examining the role of physical trauma in the onset of fibromyalgia syndrome. *Rheumatology*, 41(4), p. 450–453. https://doi.org/10.1093/rheumatology/41.4.450

Bloch, M., Schmidt, P.J., Danaceau, M., Murphy, J., Nieman, L., and Rubinow, D.R. (2000). Effects of gonadal steroids in women with a history of postpartum depression. *American Journal of Psychiatry*, 157(6), p. 924–930. https://doi.org/10.1176/appi.ajp.157.6.924

Brown, H.K., Wilton, A.S., Ray, J.G., Dennis, C.-L., Guttmann, A., and Vigod, S.N. (2019). Chronic physical conditions and risk for perinatal mental illness: A population-based retrospective cohort study. *PLOS Medicine*. https://doi.org/10.1371/journal.pmed.1002864

Caplan, P.J. (2019). Foreword. In Jo Watson (Ed), *Drop the Disorder – Challenging the Culture of Psychiatric Diagnosis*. p. xi. Monmouth, UK: PCCS Books.

Carlat, D. (2010). *Unhinged: The Trouble with Psychiatry – A Doctor's Revelations about a Profession in Crisis*. New York, London, Toronto, Sydney: Free Press.

Cohen, L.S., Altshuler, L.L., Harlow, B.L., Nonacs, R., Newport, D.J., and Viguera, A.C., et al. (2006). Relapse of major depression during pregnancy in women who maintain or discontinue antidepressant treatment. *JAMA*, 295(5), p. 499–507. https://doi.org/10.1001/jama.295.5.499

Chojenta, C., William, J., Martin, M.A., Byles, J., and Loxton, D. (2019). The impact of a history of poor mental health on health care costs in the perinatal period. *Archives of Women's Mental Health*, 22(4), p. 467–473. https://doi.org/10.1007/s00737-018-0912-4

Davies, J. (2013). *Cracked – Why Psychiatry Is Doing More Harm Than Good*. London: Icon Books.

Di Florio, A., Forty, L., Gordon-Smith, K., Heron, J., Jones, L., Craddock, N., and Jones, I. (2013). Perinatal episodes across the mood disorder spectrum. *JAMA Psychiatry*, 70, p. 168–175. https://doi.org/10.1001/jamapsychiatry.2013.279

Furness, P.J., Vogt, K., Ashe, S., Taylor, S., Haywood-Small, S., and Lawson, K. (2018). What causes fibromyalgia? An online survey of patient perspectives. *Health Psychology Open*. https://doi.org/10.1177/2055102918802683

Galvez-Sánchez, C.M., Duschek, S., and Reyes Del Paso, G.A. (2019). Psychological impact of fibromyalgia: Current perspectives. *Psychology Research and Behavior Management*, 12, p. 117–127. https://doi.org/10.2147/PRBM.S178240

Haynes, E. (2019) *"Hear Us Speak" – Listening to women's experiences of perinatal distress and the transactional analysis psychotherapy treatment they received*. PhD thesis. http://usir.salford.ac.uk/id/eprint/51465/

Irigaray, L. (1985). *The Sex Which Is Not One*. New York: Cornell University Press.

Kirsch, I. (2010). *The Emperor's New Drugs: Exploding the Antidepressant Myth*. New York: Basic Books.

Matevosyan, N.R. (2011). Pregnancy and postpartum specifics in women with schizophrenia: A meta-study. *Archives of Gynecology and Obstetrics*, 283(2), p. 141–147. https://doi.org/10.1007/s00404-010-1706-8

Moncrieff, J. (2009/2020). *A Straight Talking Introduction to Psychiatric Drugs – The Truth about How They Work and How to Come off Them* (second edition). Monmouth, UK: PCCS Books.

Schaverien, J. (2015). *Boarding School Syndrome: The Psychological Trauma of the 'Privileged' Child*. United Kingdom: Taylor & Francis.

Schiller, C.E., Meltzer-Brody, S., and Rubinow, D.R. (2015). The role of reproductive hormones in postpartum depression. *CNS Spectrums*, 20(1), p. 48–59. https://doi.org/10.1017/S1092852914000480

Timimi, S. (2020). *Insane Medicine – How the Mental Health Industry Creates Damaging Treatment Traps and How You Can Escape Them*. Self-Published.

Waszczuk, M.A., Zimmerman, M., Ruggero, C., Li, K., MacNamara, A., Weinberg, A., Hajcak, G., Watson, D., and Kotov, R. (2017). What do clinicians treat: Diagnoses or symptoms? The incremental validity of a symptom-based, dimensional characterization of emotional disorders in predicting medication prescription patterns. *Comprehensive Psychiatry*, 79, p. 80–88. https://doi.org/10.1016/j.comppsych.2017.04.004

Wesseloo, R., Kamperman, A.M., Munk-Olsen, T., Pop, V.J., Kushner, S.A., and Bergink, V. (2016). Risk of postpartum relapse in bipolar disorder and postpartum psychosis: A systematic review and meta-analysis. *American Journal of Psychiatry*, 173, p. 117–127. https://doi.org/10.1176/appi.ajp.2015.15010124

12 Affect Regulation

Introduction

The ability to self-regulate is fundamental, and yet it would seem to be one of the most common missing factors in our understanding of mental illness and particularly of maternal mental illness. A poor ability to self-regulate causes difficulties in a multitude of ways. Helping a mother, father and partner to develop their capacity to self-regulate is also fundamental in their role as caregiver to their infant. This begins with the parent literally regulating the infant, as the newborn infant has absolutely no capacity to do this for themselves. If a parent has no capacity to regulate themselves, then their ability to regulate their infant may be seriously hampered. If the essential task in the first year of human life is to create a secure attachment between infant and caregiver, then a parent who struggles with their own attachment may well then struggle with helping their infant to attach. This does not mean the parent cannot change their own ability to regulate their emotions, as Alan Schore says:

> *Although early relationships shape the developing brain, the human brain remains plastic and capable of learning throughout the entire lifespan, and with the right therapeutic help we can move beyond dissociation as our primary defence mechanism and begin to regulate our emotions more appropriately.*
>
> (Schore, 2019, p. 241–242)

Affect regulation is the ability humans have to modulate or control our emotions and the way in which they are expressed. The theory of affect regulation is nothing new, in fact, Aristotle was probably the first philosopher to highlight the importance of affects, particularly the way in which our pleasure is connected to our affective experience (Gosling & Taylor, 1982; Jurist, 1998; Stocker & Hegeman, 1996). Affects – their role and importance have been much disputed through the ages, and still are. As a clinician, affects are within the therapeutic space, between myself and my client. They are closely tied to our drives and our responses to the world around us.

DOI: 10.4324/9781003154891-14

They are crucial to our survival and also to our well-being. In psychological terms, affects are viewed in terms of the regulation of the self, by the self. Yet, once we develop regulation, it needs to be maintained, which is difficult even for the most capable of us. Affects are highly complex; we can often not know what we feel. Sometimes we may feel different things at the same time. We can also be deceived, thinking we feel one thing when actually feeling something else entirely. An example of this might be a draconian/macho father who won't let his son cry, so the son uses anger (an emotion he is allowed) instead.

When we are talking about affect regulation in psychotherapy, we are talking about the ability to regulate the self *by* our own self (self-regulation). (For an in-depth review on self-regulation, please see Burman, Green & Shanker, 2015.) As a clinician, my fundamental role is to help a client gain self-regulation and learn how to maintain it. In maternal mental illness, this is often an expansive role. If I can help the mother/father gain a semblance of regulation, I can help them, in turn, to regulate their infant, which will help the infant also to learn self-regulation. Self-regulation is a fundamental element in the caregivers' role, in turn modelling it for the child. At present, in scientific research, there is a debate over the processes which play a part in the growth and evolution of the ability we have to regulate our affect. Is it an evolutionary process or is it a biological process, and to what extent is affect regulation affected by both? Within the psychotherapy world, the work of Allan Schore has been fundamental in our ability to understand and conceptualise how important the role of affect regulation is and how treatment of mental illness may revolve around increasing our ability for this regulation.

What are affects?

Affects are our emotions. Dependent upon the philosophy a person adheres to, affects may be thought of in two separate ways. For those who are highly cognitive and adhere to logic, then the ideal would be one in which affects are integrated into cognition (Fonagy et al., 2004). The other philosophical tradition would be one in which affects were completely unconnected to, independent of, and out of control of rational thought (Fonagy et al., 2004). A philosophical debate on the historical perspectives of affects is outside the scope of this book. The stance taken here is of the absolute importance of affects – due to the fundamental role they play within the infant-caregiver bond, which is in itself an affective bond. The intensity of the bond between infant and caregiver is one of all feelings and emotional states from love through to anger, rage and terror if one is anxious about the loss of an attachment bond. Affect regulation is important from birth through to the end of life. What an infant is taught about affect regulation in infancy tends to stay with them throughout their life. Changing this ability to regulate is difficult and for those with attachment difficulties, may seem impossible. What Schore has discovered in his research is that

> *attachment promotes self-regulation and [...] this emergent function in turn allows new and more complex and resilient relational interactions between the individual and the social environment. From infancy throughout all later stages of the life span, spontaneous, rapidly acting emotional processes are centrally involved in enabling the organism to regulate and thereby cope with stresses and challenges, thus resulting in emotional resilience and well-being.*
>
> (Schore, 2019)

This evolution of ability to self-regulate from birth through to end of life and the role it then plays in our resilience to cope with everything life throws at us, is for me, the most fundamental part of working with parents. This is a relational dynamic. Every element of self-regulation originates in the fundamental first relationship an infant has with its caregivers. Helping parents to understand their role in this process and the effect it may have for their child's mental health throughout life has become one of the most important parts for me as a psychotherapist, as well as the formation of functioning healthy relationships.

There has been a huge expansion of research now into developmental neuroscience, such that we now know how fundamental attachment interactions are in the earliest of years (from the third trimester of pregnancy through to around 2 years of age) for the maturation of the brain. According to Schore (2019), the infant's brain is developing around 40,000 new synapses every second of its life and 1 million new neural connections (Center on the Developing Child, 2007). In fact, the first year of life is by far the most rapid growth and development of the brain of any time in a person's life (Kretschmann et al., 1986). It is also clear that the experiences an infant has will have an effect on the quality of their brain development. Through a process of prolific growth, then systematic pruning, the circuitry of the brain becomes more efficient. More complicated structural change happens after more simple circuits are built (Center on the Developing Child, 2007). Repeated abuse, chronic stress, neglect and severe mental illness in the mother will all have a deleterious effect on the brain development in the infant due to the lack of protection that is offered by a supportive, caring adult presence. Maternal mental illness is, therefore, a problem for the infant and not only for the mother.

What is affect regulation?

Affect regulation is fundamental as it allows us to cope with, control and modulate extremes of emotion, such as traumatic experiences and to calm ourselves allowing us to keep logical and to cope with whatever the experience is. This type of ability to regulate ourselves is learned through our interaction with those who care for us, moving from a state of co-regulation as an infant to one of self-regulation. It is developmental rather than an innate ability that some are born with and others not. Without this ability to regulate our emotions, life can seem full of anxiety, small issues can seem terrifying, leading some people to continually catastrophise. For others, they may feel constantly low and depressed, as if life is something dark and negative, with little to look forward to. It is my belief that a person's ability to regulate their affect is fundamental to a functional existence. Without this ability, many people may be prone to mental health disorders such as anxiety, distress, stress and/or depression. External factors, of course, may be used as facilitators of regulation, too, such as music, alcohol and cigarettes. However, affect regulation essentially means the regulation of the self by the self. However, it is clear that this is not the whole story.

On a basic level, in infancy, regulation is the role of the caregiver, therefore, it is a dyadic system of co-regulation with infant and caregiver, both core parts of the regulatory system. When an infant is distressed, for whatever reason, the infant cries. When that cry is attended to and the infant is calmed and soothed, they stop crying, and in the first few weeks after birth, the infant goes back to sleep. Over time, each time the infant's needs are attended to and their distress is soothed, the infant slowly learns how it is possible to calm themselves. Therefore, the regulatory system becomes individual – self-regulation. A child who has attentive parenting, whose needs are met with care, rather than drama and discord, will slowly learn over the years how to regulate themselves and how to cope with difficult experiences. In this way, affect regulation is hinged upon early relationships and, in particular, the nature of those relations.

Human beings are hugely complex, and their brains are a source of wonder. Briefly, in the 1960s, Paul MacLean created the evolutionary model of the Triune Brain (MacLean, 1990). Although this is now rejected by neuroscience due to its oversimplification, it is nevertheless a useful way of us thinking about how the brain might assess sensory information: with the Reptilian or Primal Brain (Basal Ganglia) in charge of our primal instincts, the first development; the Paleomammalian or Emotional Brain (Limbic System) in charge of our emotions or affective system, the second development; and the Neomammalian or Rational Brain (Neocortex) in charge of rational or objective thought, the final part of the brain to evolve. Affect regulation occurs in the Limbic Brain, the part that is in charge of our emotions and affective system.

We each have within us an autonomic system whose role it is to keep the body finely tuned. It is the job of our hypothalamus to coordinate the body's autonomic responses and to keep the body in a state of homeostasis. Homeostasis, in this instance, is referring to the body's self-regulating process of maintaining stability in the fundamental biological processes. Homeostasis is a dynamic system of stability (Britannica, 2021), and what this means is that the body is continuously monitoring and changing different elements of our internal processes in order to keep an equilibrium state. This equilibrium is about survival. If the body is out of equilibrium, then survival may be compromised. So, it is a fundamental part of our anatomy, yet it is something we do not know or may have no idea is happening. It is just there, in our bodies, all the time. Affect regulation plays a role in homeostasis. The hypothalamus is constantly monitoring our body's different parameters (for example, temperature, heart rate and glucose levels), bringing them back to their optimal position as soon as they deviate. The hypothalamus coordinates the body's autonomic responses and gains its information from the limbic system as well as from higher brain structures like the neocortex. The body always strives for homeostasis – the body's pull to remain in a stabilised state with physiological constancy and a steady state equilibrium. When the body is pulled out of homeostasis, the hypothalamus very quickly mounts a strong response – because being out of homeostasis threatens our whole being. The response is three-fold – engaging the autonomic nervous system, the endocrine system and the behavioural system. When distress occurs, the body is pulled out of homeostasis and the hypothalamus gets to action to try and bring it back to equilibrium again.

The hypothalamus takes in all sorts of information from the external and internal environment, from our internal organs, blood pressure levels and hormones. It controls our circadian rhythms, and it is also affected by stress and changes in cortisol (the stress hormone). It produces excitatory and inhibitory hormones which stop and start other hormone release within the body. It is thought to be the link between the endocrine system and the nervous system. The hypothalamus is possibly the most important part of the endocrine system, as it alerts the pituitary gland to release hormones into the rest of the endocrine system, keeping the internal processes of the body in balance and in check.

The body likes to remain in homeostasis. However, if a person grew up in an environment that was distressing or unsafe, that child may feel stressed or fearful for a large proportion of their life. Within their body, they are likely to be releasing large levels of cortisol and adrenaline. What might the effect of these neurotransmitters be on human?

Why is affect regulation so important?

For the first 6 months of an infant's life, emotions appear to be totally dependent upon how the caregiver responds to the child. After 6 months, the emotions become subjective for the infant and become about the caregiver's attitude to the infant, how they behave with the infant and how accessible they are to the infant's needs. The infant is only operating at this stage with its amygdala. The hippocampus has not yet developed and formed properly, so all stimuli and responses to those stimuli are processed through the amygdala, laying down critical emotional memories which are beyond our conscious awareness. Key affective and relational patterns are encoded and stored in the infant's developing brain. It is these primary, implicit experiences of self and other that combine to form our life positions (how we view ourselves as opposed to others – such as I am not OK as there is something fundamentally wrong with me, but all others are OK). These experiences at this early age are not necessarily pathological and are more about the infant making sense of their life with important 'others'. These experiences do begin to interfere with a child's ability to generate new relational possibilities, however. At this early age, the child stores sensorimotor patterns or schemas containing all the first emotional reactions that shaped our lives as small infants, such as bodily postures. These are often non-narratable and are felt in the body. They may be intense patterns of relating which are not accessible to memory, story or narrative. As such, they will be the experiences that sit beneath many trans-ferential experiences – impasses, enactments, parallel processes and projective identification, for example. They are often touched or triggered in our most intimate relationships, at a point of both hope and dread. When these are triggered, they can bring the most intense anxiety and can feel almost impos-sible to tolerate, understand and resolve.

Dependent upon whether affect-regulation and indeed affects themselves are seen from a psychoanalytic perspective or an attachment theory perspective the views may be different. Attachment theorists believe that secure attach-ment equals good affect regulation. Psychoanalysts see affects as primitive, powerful forces linked to motivation and drive theory. As such, they may be out of our awareness or indeed unconscious forces, yet affect regulation is seen as also important for psychoanalysts. Fonagy et al. take the concept of affect regulation forwards to a sense of self-regulation, achieved through affects, but also beyond just affects. '*In one sense, self-regulation can be considered as a higher kind of affect regulation; in another sense, it constitutes a change in form*' (2004, p. 95). By this, they mean allowing the affect to be felt for self-understanding, as well as for more cognitive reasons – the appraisal, informational processing and attention towards the affects. In so doing, having the capability of (choosing to) change the emotional state or not adjusting it at all bringing in a reflective function – mentalization – which allows for a new relationship with our own affects. In Transactional Analysis, this may be viewed as the integrating Adult ego state (Tudor, 2003) – the ability to self-regulate whilst in the affective state. This is not an easy position to achieve, as it is so easy to mistake our feelings and to misunderstand them.

In Figure 12.1, I am showing the very first months of an infant's life and the role of the caregiver. In the very first few weeks after birth, the infant spends the majority of its time asleep. During wakefulness, it is in one of two states – distress (crying), or brief moments of awareness, primary consciousness (Stern, 1985), when the infant's eyes are open, but they are unable to focus on things around them, other than possibly if they are being fed or are close enough to make out another. Stern talks about an infant having the capacity to differ-entiate self from other at birth and that this is 'in place and in process almost from the very beginning' (p. xiii). Taipale also talks about '*The pressing need organizes the infant's whole experiential reality, and the caregiver is initially nothing more than what she is in the light of the infant's current needs and wants*' (2016b).

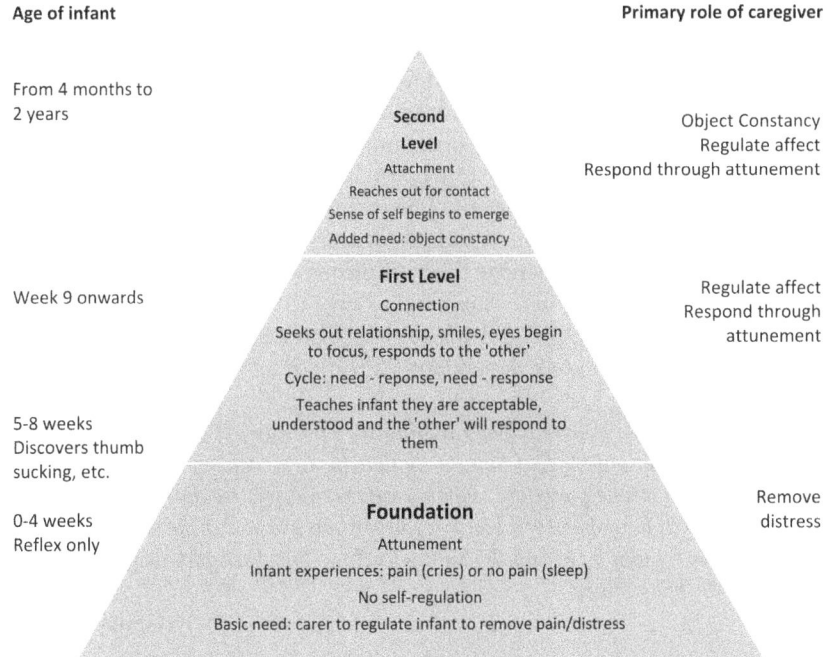

Age of infant

From 4 months to
2 years

Week 9 onwards

5-8 weeks
Discovers thumb
sucking, etc.

0-4 weeks
Reflex only

Primary role of caregiver

Second
Level
Attachment
Reaches out for contact
Sense of self begins to emerge
Added need: object constancy

Object Constancy
Regulate affect
Respond through attunement

First Level
Connection
Seeks out relationship, smiles, eyes begin
to focus, responds to the 'other'
Cycle: need - reponse, need - response
Teaches infant they are acceptable,
understood and the 'other' will respond to
them

Regulate affect
Respond through
attunement

Foundation
Attunement
Infant experiences: pain (cries) or no pain (sleep)
No self-regulation
Basic need: carer to regulate infant to remove pain/distress

Remove
distress

Figure 12.1 First three levels of an infant's needs and the role of the primary caregiver

Piontelli goes one step further and suggests that fetuses may also have a sem-blance of awareness of the me/not me (Piontelli, 1992), which she attributes to '*a remarkable continuity in aspects of pre-natal and post-natal life*' (p. 1).

I call the very first few weeks after birth 'Foundation', which I see as a time for the parents to learn to attune to their infant, with the infant's basic needs of regulation and the removal of pain/distress. Those first few weeks are seemingly about rest and recuperation after the experience of being born and adaptation to their new environment. They have the startle reflex and the grasp reflex at this point in their development, and the new world around them may seem loud and full in comparison to the environment in the womb, where the light is dim, and other things remain constant such as temperature. They can hear noise in the womb, but it will be muffled.

> *The affective environment of the infant is multifarious and overwhelming, and if the sensory-affective external environment of the infant would not be organized by keeping an eye on her deficient affective regulative capacities, the infant would be injured by the overwhelming stimuli.*
>
> (Taipale, 2016a)

There is also a correlation between the way in which glucose is utilized in the brain and behavioural and neurophysiological maturation (Chugani &

Phelps, 1986). In the first month, the brain is utilising glucose in the sensori-motor part of the brain. When an infant is distressed, this may be due to the experience of a feeling which the infant may never have felt before, such as a dirty nappy, hunger or fear from a loud noise, for example, all of which may seem overwhelming to a newly born infant. They need reassurance which may be through cuddling and touch, rocking and gentle talking to them. This reassurance is very important. The parent's role is to manage the infant's regulation. An infant who is constantly distressed and hyperaroused in these earliest of weeks cannot manage their emotions at all and will be totally reliant on the carer to respond to them and to give them what they need to calm and soothe them enough to go back to sleep again. An infant in these earliest weeks of birth is absolutely dependent (Winnicott, 1965).

> *Physiologically, the human baby is still very much part of the mother's body. He depends on her milk to feed him, to regulate his heart rate and blood pressure, and to provide immune protection. His muscular activity is regulated by her touch, as is his growth hormone level. Her body keeps him warm and she disperses his stress hormones for him by her touch and her feeding. This basic physiological regulation keeps the baby alive.*

(Gerhardt, 2004)

This affect regulation is verbal and non-verbal, done by the voice, the rocking of the baby, the holding, the touch and the attention. It is a bodily action as well as a verbal one. An infant is highly sensitive to these verbal and non-verbal messages. These then become what Daniel Stern calls Representations of Interactions that have been Generalised (RIGs) (1985). These RIGs then are indelibly held in the brain at an unconscious level and form part of our patterns of behaviour within our relationships for the rest of our life. Even at this stage, an infant may have a very rudimentary way of self-regulation. They will instinctively turn away from stimuli that is too much (Gergely & Watson, 1996), and of course, some babies very early on learn to self soothe through thumb or hand sucking.

The second stage, from about 2 months onwards, I call 'first level' which is a level of connection and is when an infant begins to communicate with others. They are gradually attaching to the caregiver, which we can begin to see by the infant smiling at those they recognise, and responding by wiggling their body and synchronously moving their arms when the caregiver talks to them to show their pleasure in the other (Trevarthen & Aitken, 2001). The infant will begin to look for and favour the caregiver and will find new people strange and at first frightening and look for reassurance from the caregiver that this strange person is OK.

The brain begins to take up glucose into the parietal, temporal and primary visual cortices (Franceschini et al., 2007). This makes sense as this is the stage when we begin to notice that the infant is able to see better, they seem to see the parent and begin to smile in recognition, as well as verbalising by normally cooing and gurgling, and they may also seem to be trying to copy mouth actions. They may briefly calm themselves by sucking on their hand or mouth when they find them, which may provide brief comfort. But they cannot mitigate too much sound and may find sudden noise quite frightening. It is up to the caregiver to respond to their fear, their startle and their discomfort. The carer will be managing their regulation. At this point, the infant will turn their head towards sounds, and they will begin to follow things with their eyes. As their eyesight becomes clearer, they may begin to recognize people at more of a distance. They can also show their boredom and may begin to fuss if they are left without stimulation or if their activity is not changed often. Finally, they are more able to hold their head up and can begin to push up on their arms a little when they are left on their tummy. This is a time when the caregiver needs to regulate affect as well as respond through attunement and is the beginning of the infant learning the need-response cycle. At the outset, the infant is totally dependent upon the caregiver to manage their regulation. Through time and a good, responsive caregiver, there is a subtle shift towards the parent 'assisting' the infant to regulate, where the infant slowly experiences and is able to cope with small levels of dysregulation which she is able to manage with the assistance of the parent, rather than the parent managing the regulation for her.

From 4 months onwards, the infant is in the second level where they have the capacity to smile spontaneously and will laugh. In brain development terms, glucose uptake is now increasing in the lateral inferior frontal cortex (Franceschini et al., 2007). Their communication skills improve, and many infants begin to babble as their language and communication skills are built. The sound they make when they cry also may become much more nuanced so that the parent can often determine whether they are hungry, tired or in pain. The infant can now reach out for contact, from a parent, for a toy that is in reach. They begin to gain strength in their muscles and begin to move through rolling and can push up higher when on their tummy. They can often hold a toy and shake it or put it towards their mouth. This is when they begin to learn hand–eye coordination and can reach for a toy they can see, as well as follow things that are moving in front of them so that the capacity to move their eyes from side to side is now there. The parent's role builds on the responding through attunement and affect regulation into one of becoming the needed constant object so that the infant feels safe and secure. This is the time when the infant will show their recognition of people and will seem to be watching faces very closely. They have no ability yet to speak, but this is the beginning of them trying to make sense of what is going on. Very much by repetition, by mirroring actions, sounds, gestures and by being engaged in the infant, the infant is learning how the mother responds and engages with them. It is at this point that engagement in the infant is so important.

We know that when a mother disengages from her baby through Tronick's famous 'still face experiment' (Tronick et al., 1975) that very quickly the baby becomes extremely distressed and dysregulated. The baby is expecting feedback from the mother, the mirroring that the mother has always done and that is so natural between mother and infant, so when there is no response from the mother but her face remains still and impassive, it would appear that the infant is confused and tries very hard to invite the parent back into relationship and connection. We can imagine that when a mother is very unwell with maternal mental illness and has little capacity to engage with her baby that the baby will eventually give up 'inviting' the mother into connection. There is little or no mirroring and the infant is left in a void where they are not recognized and as if the infant is not there or does not exist. The infant is not able to learn how they feel through the mirroring mother continuously repeating the mirroring back of emotion.

We know that at 6 months of age, a baby is able to know whether a person is strange or familiar. They are becoming very well attached to their parents by now and will like to play, interact and remain connected as a form of safety and security. They are able to respond to others' emotions and may be fascinated with looking at themselves in a mirror. Brain development by 1 year is in the dorsal and medial frontal cortex (Franceschini et al., 2007).

Sroufe (1996) describes a system whereby emotions are experienced subjectively. In the first 6 months of life, the infant's regulation is dependent upon how the caregiver responds to the infant and what they do with that infant's distress. From 6 months onwards, Sroufe believes that emotions begin to become subjective for the infant and become about the caregiver's attitude to the infant, how they behave with the infant and how accessible they are to the infant's needs (1996). Thus, from a developmental sense, it is the interaction between infant and caregiver and the infant's subjective experience of that caregiver that shapes the infant's affective experience (Fonagy et al., 2004). Taipale (2016a) agrees that we are impacted by others, by their *subjectivity (i.e. their intentions, gestures, perceptions, reactions, moods, attitudes, emotional expressions, verbal reports, etc.), and we tend to be particularly sensitive when their experiences are directed at us'*. This helps us to understand that also others continue to regulate us, and the way we are perceived by others, particularly those who know us well, can continue to influence our behaviour, in the form of co-regulation. We each have an implicit memory system, which is how we interact with others and the rules around this that we learned at a very early age. Let's think of an infant who is afraid, yet the caregiver does not know what the infant is afraid of. The response of the carer is vital. A kind, loving and understanding response from a carer who acknowledges the child's fear and who calms and soothes the infant helps the child to move onto something else, acknowledging the fear yet helping the infant see that life moves on and these fears subside. This is a very different experience to a child who is told to stop being a cry-baby, whose fear is not recognised and is ignored. That child learns that fear is not acceptable and needs to be hidden in whatever way possible.

> *What the infant internalizes in the earliest developmental stages is destined to largely outline her capacities in affective self-regulation.*

> (Taipale, 2016a)

In terms of their interpersonal relationships, infants are learning a non-symbolic representational system which the Boston Change Study Group calls '*implicit relational knowing*' (Lyons-Ruth et al., 1998). Implicit relational knowing '*encompasses normal and pathological knowings and integrates affect, fantasy, behavioural, and cognitive dimensions*' (Lyons-Ruth et al., 1998, p. 284). This is a non-verbal procedural representation of how to proceed, how to do things, and in particular, how to do things with others. This would include many different things such as how to gain attention from others in childhood, how to show affection to others, and how to be with others generally. Lyons-Ruth emphasises that these knowings are '*as much affective and interactive as they are cognitive*' (p. 284). This all occurs prior to language and then continues and stays with us for the rest of our lives. We do not know we have learnt this, as it is non-conscious. Yet it is something that is co-constructed between us and our parents/caregivers and continues to be adapted and updated throughout life. What is important to understand is that the capacity to differentiate pleasure from non-pleasure and to further categorise these into specific affective states/emotions is actually a developmental achievement, as is the ability to become self-reflective about those states. Unless someone has received this level of mirroring and good enough parenting from the beginning, through all the developmental stages which allow the infant to gradually learn social referencing and to internalize affect mirroring and regulation, this person will not be able to regulate their own affect in the way that is helpful and healthy for them in their life. This person is, therefore, likely to become dysregulated easily and will continue to seek and need regulation from another. For the many women I see with maternal mental illness who come into therapy in a state of hyperarousal and with high levels of distress, I know that these women, at this moment, do not have the capacity to regulate their own affects. Therefore, a form of therapeutic co-regulation needs to be the priority in our therapeutic role.

References

Britannica. (2021). https://www.britannica.com/science/homeostasis [accessed 05.11.21].

Burman, J.T., Green, C.D., and Shanker, S. (2015). On the meanings of self-regulation: Digital humanities in service of conceptual clarity, *Child Development*, 86(5), p.1507–1521. https://doi.org/10.1111/cdev.12395

Center on the Developing Child. (2007). *The Science of Early Childhood Development* (In Brief). Retrieved from www.developingchild.harvard.edu [accessed 05.11.21].

Chugani, H.T., and Phelps, M.E. (1986). Maturational changes in cerebral function in infants determined by 18FDG positron emission tomography. *Science,* 231(4740), p 840–843. https://doi.org/10.1126/science.3945811

Fonagy, P., Gergely, G., Jurist, E.L., and Targe, M. (2004). *Affect Regulation, Mentalization, and Development of the Self.* New York: Other Press.

Franceschini, M.A., Thaker, S., Themelis, G., Krishnamoorthy, K.K., Bortfeld, H., Diamond, S.G., Boas, D.A., Arvin, K., and Grant, E. (2007). Assessment of infant brain development with frequency-domain near-infrared spectroscopy. *Pediatric Research,* 61(5), p. 546–551. https://doi.org/10.1203/pdr.0b013e318045be99

Gergely, G., and Watson, J.S. (1996). The social biofeedback theory of parental affect-mirroring: The development of emotional self-awareness. *The International Journal of Psychoanalysis,* 77, p. 1181–1212.

Gerhardt, S. (2004). *Why Love Matters: How Affection Shapes a Baby's Brain.* Hove, East Sussex: Routledge.

Gosling, J.C.B., and Taylor, C.C.W. (1982). *The Greeks on Pleasure.* Oxford: Clarendon Press.

Jurist, E. (1998). The unexamined life is not worth living: Michael Stocker on emotions. *Metaphilosophy,* 29, p. 223–231.

Kretschmann, H.J., Kammradt, G., Krauthausen, I., Sauer, B., and Wingert, F. (1986). Brain growth in man. *Bibliotheca Anatomica,* (28), p. 1–26. PMID: 3707509.

Lyons-Ruth, K., Bruschweiler-Stern, N., Harrison, A.M., Morgan, A., Nahum, J.P., Sander, L., Stern, D.N., Tronick, E.Z. (1998). Implicit Relational Knowing: Its Role in Development and Psychoanalytic Treatment. Infant Mental Health Journal, 19(3), p. 282–289

MacLean, P.D. (1990). *The Triune Brain in Evolution: Role in Paleocerebral Functions.* New York: Springer

Piontelli, A. (1992). *From Fetus to Child: An Observational and Psychoanalytic Study.* East Sussex: Brunner-Routledge.

Schore, A. (2019). *Right Brain Psychotherapy.* New York: W.W. Norton & Company.

Sroufe, L. (1996). *Emotional Development: The Organization of Emotional Life in Early Years.* New York: Cambridge University Press.

Stern, D.N. (1985). *The Interpersonal World of the Infant: A View from Psychoanalysis and Developmental Psychology.* New York: Basic Books.

Stocker, M., and Hegeman, E. (1996). *Valuing Emotions.* Cambridge, UK: Cambridge University Press.

Taipale, J. (2016a). Self-regulation and beyond: Affect regulation and the infant-caregiver dyad. *Frontiers in Psychology,* 7, p. 889. https://doi.org/10.3389/fpsyg.2016.00889

Taipale, J. (2016b). The pain of granting otherness. Interoception and the emergence of the object. In R.T. Jensen & D. Moran (Eds), *The Phenomenology of Embodied Subjectivity.* p. 241–262. Dordrecht: Springer.

Trevarthen, C., and Aitken, K. (2001) Infant intersubjectivity: Research, theory, and clinical applications. *Journal of Child Psychology and Psychiatry,* 42, p. 3–48. https://doi.org/10.1111/1469-7610.00701

Tronick, E., Adamson, I., Als, H., and Brazelton, T. (1975). Infant emotion in normal and pertubated interactions. *Paper presented at the Biennial Meeting of the Society for Research in Child Development,* Denver, CO.

Tudor, K. (2003). The neopsyche: The integrating adult ego state. In C. Sills & H. Hargaden (Eds), *Ego states (Vol. 1 of Key Concepts in Transactional Analysis: Contemporary Views).* p. 201–231. London: Worth Publishing.

Winnicott, D. (1965). *The Maturational Processes and the Facilitating Environment: Studies in the Theory of Emotional Development.* New York: International Universities Press.

13 The Therapeutic Role

This chapter explores our therapeutic role as relational psychotherapists. I see our role as being similar to the role of the parent with their newborn infant. Whereby, there will be emotionally charged encounters, much as there will be with a small infant. However, our ability as therapists to regulate our client's emotional self-states is crucial for the process of change within psychotherapy. Schore (2019) describes this as the '*therapist's right brain visual-facial, auditory-prosodic, and tactile-gestural capacities for the nonverbal communication*'. What he means by this is that we are using the right hemisphere of our brain to engage with the right hemisphere of our client's brain, through nonverbal, unconscious emotional, and relational communication. This is as opposed to left brain conscious cognition.

I have included a similar diagram to the one in Chapter 6, but in this instance, it shows the primary, secondary and tertiary functions of psychotherapy within maternal mental illness, which I see as a focus on:

- Reducing the woman's distress
- The need for attachment in therapy and how this will be similar to the client's original attachment style
- Object constancy

These three elements begin to build the needed relationship with our client, and help the client to feel listened to, attuned and attended to. It is these elements that help to form an implicit, safe enough, relational environment within which the client can start to feel, contact, describe and then learn to regulate their own subjective experience. These elements help our clients to feel safe enough to then form a narrative about what has happened to them. Once we hear their narrative, this then becomes, of itself, a way of marking change within the therapeutic relationship. This is not an interpretation of narrative, as interpretation is cognitive. This is much more than that. Often the narrative has remained unspoken for years and builds a charge within the person. It can cause rumination, anxiety, shame, guilt, all the emotions which continue the cycle of dysregulation. Being able to speak their narrative

DOI: 10.4324/9781003154891-15

allows their story to be out in the world. It gives a sense of realness, that their story is witnessed. This telling and then seeing and hearing the response of the therapist changes the story into an interpersonal experience, one in which the client then receives verbal and nonverbal responses. Regulation occurs interpersonally, from one brain to another brain: '*the self-organization of the developing brain occurs in the context of a relationship with another self, another brain*' (Schore, 1996, p. 60). Once the client is able to sufficiently regulate themselves then there is the ability to grow and engender a secure sense of self: emotional well-being on an interpersonal intersubjective level as well as an intrapersonal intrapsychic level. What we are attempting to do is to help a client build their capacity for reflective function so that they can improve their ability to remain in their emotion and yet keep one foot out of the emotion as such, to anchor them to the present moment. This enables the woman to feel her emotion, and also retain her reflective capacity and be curious about what she is feeling and why this might be. This is similar to a mother feeling her infant's emotion and yet still remaining curious and open about this emotion, whilst nonetheless calming and soothing her infant. The infant's emotion does not overpower the mother. She can instead transform the emotion into something more palatable for the infant by attuning to and then soothing and calming the infant. In psychotherapeutic terms we call this transformational transference (Ogden, 1982/1992). Here, I am using Ogden's idea that the infant will 'project' a feeling state into the mother/carer that is similar to the feeling that the infant is not able to process for themselves and may therefore feel intolerable to the infant. This is a process called projective identification when it occurs as a transferential element in the therapy relationship. What is important is the carer's ability to transform the infant's feeling into something more palatable for the infant, something the infant is able to bear. This is replicated in the transferential interaction between therapist and client where the client experiences the therapist as turning her intolerable feelings into something more palatable.

The therapeutic alliance

One of the most important things in psychotherapy, regardless of modality, is the therapeutic alliance. There is now empirical evidence to show this (Horvath & Symonds, 1991; Martin, Garske & Davis, 2000) and how it functions as part of the change process. There is also research on the predictive relationship, rupture, and repair in the relationship, and also the validity of training psychotherapists to improve the therapeutic alliance through focusing on their interpersonal relationship with their client (see Muran & Barber, 2010 for a fuller description). There is no doubt that the alliance between client and therapist is fundamental for the therapy to be successful. What is therefore important is for psychotherapists to focus on the relationship they have with their clients, and to understand that this will have a predictive capacity on the success or failure of the therapy (Paley & Lawton, 2001).

How do we fulfil this need to focus on the therapeutic alliance or on the relational dyad if you wish to call it that? And what is our therapeutic role with women who are struggling with maternal mental illness?

Our therapeutic role

When a client comes to therapy, they will most often arrive distressed. Some will know why they are distressed; others will not, as it will be outside their conscious awareness. I see my primary role as helping them alleviate the distress they feel, in order to be better able to use therapy for whatever it is they want to achieve, which is most often change. When a person remains distressed, it is difficult to get them to focus on anything other than their distress, and so for me it is vital that I help them to find a way to calm and soothe themselves. What is clear from neuroscientific research is that distress (stress, anxiety, trauma, etc.) will change the function of the brain, and may in fact change the structure of the brain in areas such as the hypothalamus, basal ganglia, the cingulate cortex and the insula. These areas are all associated with greater anxiety, post-traumatic stress disorder (PTSD) symptoms, distress and depression. Therefore, it is important to find a way to help the client alleviate their distress from the outset of therapy.

From the very first moment I am thinking about and focusing on connection and relationship. I am noticing how the client feels and I am wondering about their sense of safety and security. I know that what is also important is my own connection and relationship with myself. If I have utilised my own therapy, supervision and continuing professional development well, I will be far more able to remain client-focused, to attune to my client, and be curious about their frame of reference and how this will be impacting them negatively. Each client has a very different story and will need to be treated differently. None of the mothers and fathers I see are treated the same. I do not have a 'manualised' approach as I do not believe this helps. I know that one woman with maternal anxiety will not be the same as any other. There will be similarities, yes. But they will not be the same. Each client needs to be approached as totally new, utterly unique, and fundamentally different. My approach therefore needs to be adaptable, flexible, resourceful and creative. As research now evidences (Dreyfus & Dreyfus, 1986), flexibility in approach – which I believe needs to be specific to each client, -creativity within the approach, and focusing on my client's specific needs are the most important elements and begin in those immediate moments of meeting with a new client.

Psychotherapists need to provide an environment that is warm and caring. But this is not the whole story. Dependent upon the type of psychotherapy that is being offered, the therapist needs to be clear about what constitutes their style of psychotherapy, what the contract will be both administratively and therapeutically, and the way in which they will facilitate the client to become aware of how they are and how they live in the world so that they can begin to think differently about themselves and others. In Transactional Analysis, this is called deconfusion, which, in essence, is helping the client become less confused about what is going on both intrapsychically and interpersonally. This helps to build a client's awareness and also helps them to learn about their self-defeating or self-destructive thoughts and behaviours. Within the therapeutic alliance as far as possible there needs to be transparency, which occurs through open communication. This is vitally important so that the client and the therapist are both thinking, active participants within the process, and there is a mutuality of relationship where the intelligence and potential to contribute is equal and the responsibility for the process of therapy is joint. Mutuality means that both know what the aims and objectives of the therapy are and can then co-create a therapeutic contract together. This transparency and the bilateral nature of forming this therapeutic contract together helps both know how they are going to work together and what their respective roles and tasks are to achieve the goal. They both will also know when the client has achieved the 'goal' of therapy. And most importantly, this highlights that all people are OK and that relational therapy is not about power; it is about mutuality and equality.

The fundamental part of this is the therapeutic relationship between therapist and client: how the therapist builds a sense of collaboration and rapport through things such as empathic listening, attunement, implicit relational knowing, gentle challenge and confrontation.

The primary, secondary and tertiary functions of psychotherapy

Figure 13.1 shows an illustration of the primary, secondary and tertiary functions of psychotherapy with women with maternal mental illness.

The primary function

When a client first comes to therapy they will really want and expect the therapist to calm their distress. However, this can take quite a whilst, and it occurs through many different elements, such as paying attention to the therapeutic alliance that is building, listening and really hearing the client's story, and empathising with the client, amongst other things. The client will have an expectation that if they are not coming away feeling less distressed quickly in the therapy, the therapy is not working. Yet it takes time to get to know our clients, to begin to understand what is going on for them. It will also take time for the client to really know and understand at a deeper level, what the aim is for their therapy. This aim may well not be what the client originally came with. Quite often, we find ourselves working with elements that were unconscious or preconscious at the beginning of the work, and only come into focus through the alliance we build together. Clients will often want some form of change. It is helpful to explore and define change, focusing our attention on how change can be achieved and how the client wants the change to occur. Building trust can take time, and is about helping

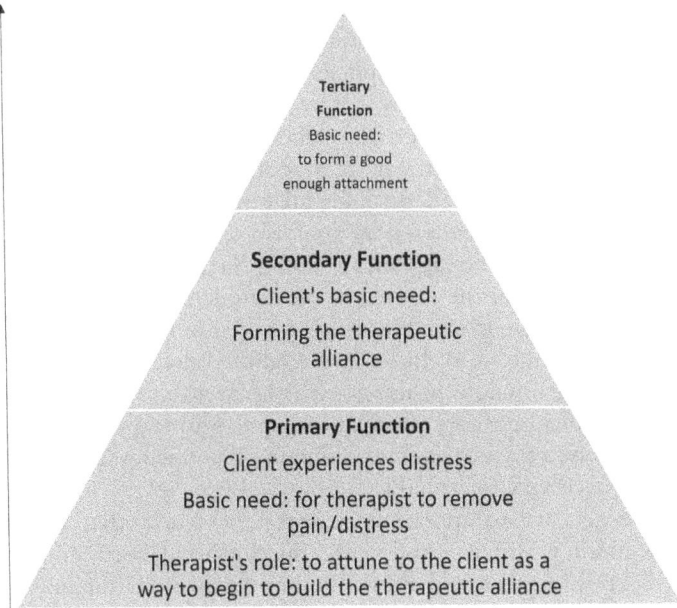

Figure 13.1 The three psychotherapeutic functions when working with maternal mental illness

to build a good enough relationship between therapist and client, so our clients begin to value the therapeutic alliance and process. Once this occurs they are likely to stay, so change can occur over the long term.

Similarly, to a mother/carer with her new infant, the primary role forms the building blocks for the next two roles. The primary role will also continue onwards and become a part of those next two roles so that each one builds upon the role below. This helps to build a strong foundation for the therapeutic alliance, something that will become important during the inevitable ruptures that will occur in the therapy.

The secondary function

The therapeutic alliance is key to the second function, which is to address the need for attachment in therapy.

> *Attachment promotes self-regulation and [...] this emergent function in turn allow new and more complex and resilient relational interactions between the individual and the social environment ... From infancy throughout all later stages of the life span, spontaneous, rapidly acting emotional processes are centrally involved in enabling the organism to regulate and thereby cope with stresses and challenges, thus resulting in emotional resilience and well-being.*
>
> (Schore, 2019, p. 158)

Attachment in therapy begins with connection and, again, similarly to the mother with her newborn, connection comes through attunement and from implicit relational knowing. Implicit relational knowing (Lyons-Ruth, 1998) is the intersubjective space between the therapist and the client in which we both sense the other, the other's needs, struggles, blind spots, emotions and as therapists we start to respond to them as they arise in the client. Attachment is formed through all our senses, not simply through narrative, although helping a client to form a narrative that is meaningful for them is crucial (Fonagy et al., 2004; Spence, 1982). An infant can perceive the emotion of the carer with no language, but with their intense gaze, and at a felt sense level, humans seem to retain the capacity to perceive the 'other' in adulthood too. In fact, in relational psychotherapy, the use of these primitive unconscious processes, which we refer to as the transferential domain, becomes important. In relational psychotherapy the belief is that the work is often in the unconscious domain. The unconscious becomes the part that it is necessary to attend to.

When we go back to attachment theory, we know that attachment is formed in infancy and is a reflection on the bond between parent and infant. We know a great deal about the importance of attachment in relationship and the positive impact this has on a person's reflective capacity (what Fonagy et al., call 'mentalization'). For a detailed description of the empirical evidence on attachment and capacity for self-reflection please see Fonagy et al. (2004). Therefore, when treating a woman with maternal mental illness we may perceive in her a lack of secure attachment, and a need for the 'other' to modulate or calm her affects, rather than her having learned the capacity for self-modulation in infancy. This is important, because in the psychotherapeutic relationship, we will find that the attachment style from infancy then becomes part of the relational dyad. It may be, for example, that the woman has never felt secure or safe, and thus providing a safe and secure environment for her to trust enough to attach to will become the first part of the 'needed' relationship between therapist and client. What we will find also is that the type of attachment will get played out within the therapeutic relationship. What I mean is that there will be a behavioural manifestation in the client which is shown through various aspects such as their interpretation of events, feelings, emotions, the way they perceive others' behaviours, and sometimes engaging in self-destructive or self-harming behaviours.

It is also very likely that the client will attach to their therapist using their only known attachment style, in much the same way as they attached to their original caregivers. The change of attachment style is an aim of therapy, with the client forming a new, trusted and secure attachment with us as their therapist. Once that is formed within the therapeutic relationship, this will model a new way of being for the client in their intimate relationships, particularly within the new mother/child dyad she has with her own child.

The tertiary function

If a client has an insecure disorganized attachment style (attachment trauma) and has experienced little in the way of safety and security through life, the third function becomes vital in the therapeutic relationship, as the therapist will need to be emotionally accessible to the client, in order to bridge the gap left by the emotionally inaccessible parent. This woman will be expecting the therapist to be inconsistent, and either intrusive or disengaged, in much the same way as her own mother may have been. Schore shows us how this will have had an impact on the right hemisphere of the brain creating '*a predisposition to emotional dysregulation and thereby psychopathology*' (Schore, 2019, p. 166). Schore has continued to express that relational trauma will cause a predisposition to '*pathological dissociation and a susceptibility to later disorders of affect regulation expressed in a deficit in coping with future socioemotional stressors*'. When a woman is highly distressed, one of the things that is important to hold loosely in our mind is what the original attachment style might have been, and what we will need to offer to our client, in order to change this style.

This third function is for the therapist to become similar to a 'constant object'. Object constancy comes from the theory of Object Relations and simply means that a person knows and understands that a relationship remains stable and will not disintegrate even if there are ruptures, setbacks, conflicts or disagreements. Many people who have had disruptive or difficult relationships in childhood will experience extreme anxiety and fear of abandonment in relationships. In fact, even some who would appear to have had an OK childhood can still fear abandonment. A lack of trust in your parents when you were a child can lead a person to struggle with issues of trust and acceptance in adulthood and will lead to them constantly needing reassurance from the other, as they are so fearful that the relationship is not permanent and the other will disappear at any moment. This is as important as it is for an infant, where the caregiver also needs to be their constant object. Again, this is part of the formation of trust in the other.

I find that many women who struggle with maternal mental illness have a sketchy sense of safety and security and this can lead to them appearing to be 'needy' in therapy. Actually, this need is vital. The woman may not vocalise why she feels in need of the therapist. However, being able to form a strong, safe attachment in therapy, with the client knowing that the therapist is there for them (in a professional capacity), can help them to form new relational patterns and habits, which will help a woman to address her own infant's need for object constancy. A mother who has never felt safe and secure may have absolutely no idea how to provide safety and security for her infant. Modelling this for her, and helping to provide her with a (professional) optimal attachment experience in therapy, will help her to begin to develop her emotional right brain and thus her capacity for resilience in stressful situations. This will also reduce her symptomatic behaviour, her intrusive thoughts, her rumination and her catastrophising. She may let go of her need to control and for her motherhood experience to be perfect in every aspect. Any obsessive-compulsive thoughts or behaviours will also begin to subside.

> *The fundamental experience of self is a right-hemispheric affair… when right-hemispheric function is diminished, so also are those features associated with the overarching concepts of self, including inhibitory control and a background state of well-being.*
> (Meares, 2012, p. 296)

When combined in therapy, these three elements begin to build the needed relationship with our client. Once we have the needed relationship, and there is a stronger element of co-regulation, we can then work towards helping the client re-formulate their thinking and emotional patterns, their relationships, their motivations and scripts and work towards them changing these for good.

The clients' narrative as a clue to change

One element of my client work I find particularly helpful is to pay attention to my client's narrative. Quite often our clients will tell us the same story many times over in many different ways. I believe this shows that the client is unable to frame their story in any other way and that they will be stuck in a particular 'impasse', or part of their story. However, after a period of time it is interesting to note that these same stories begin to subtly change. At first, the change will be so subtle that it is almost unnoticeable. However, at some point, there is an obvious change and as a therapist we can feed that back to our clients, to highlight that the client is indeed changing.

Another element of the narrative to note is the temporal change. What I mean by this is noticing the tense of the verb that a client is using, be it past, present, future, etc. At the outset clients often talk in the present or past tense. This can mean several things. Sometimes, they dwell on the past in a negative way, and it is possible to find a client almost unable to talk about the present. This may be because they are quite fixated on what happened then – back then. The way this can be framed and can feel to the therapist is that the client is almost reliving the past and continues to want to relive and replay this historical story. I believe this is because the client does not feel that the story is yet resolved. In supervision, my supervisees will often tell me that the client keeps telling the same story over and over. For me, this offers us information about the client and what is going on for them, so I believe our role is simply to observe and wonder what it is about the story that is stuck, that the client is unable to move on from, and how we might help them to do this. One way is by helping the client build their capacity for reflective functioning, to become curious about themselves, their thoughts and feelings, and what it is that brings them to this place of negativity and stuckness. Another way will be through using supervision, wondering with other therapists what might be going on for the client, using our experience and countertransference and that of our peers to help unpick the story and gain a sense of what might be happening for the client. Using supervision in this way can allow us to pool knowledge and ideas on how best to proceed with a client.

There is one other element that can be important in this stage of the therapy. Quite often a process can occur and can be played out between the mother and infant, and then between the mother and therapist. This is an important element to understand and to use, particularly with clients with little experience of a good enough mother, or a lack, such as those who lost their mother prior to childbirth.

Case example: The motherless mother

Camilla was in her early thirties and came to me when her son, Ernest, was 6 months old. She initially came to therapy because of her anxiety about Ernest and a fear that something bad would happen to him. In our assessment session, she told me that she had been referred to her perinatal mental health team but was quickly discharged by the team. Camilla's mother had committed suicide a few weeks prior to Ernest's birth. Camilla told me she was consumed with shame and guilt, believing that she could have done something to stop her mother.

Some of the prevalent themes of her therapy were:

- Terror that something bad would happen to Ernest
- Shame and guilt around her mother's suicide
- Being missed, by her parents, by her teachers, by social services, by the perinatal crisis team
- A need to mask her emotions – so no one could see how bad she felt
- Letting go

In that initial session Camilla tried to project a persona of competency. This continued each week, with her always seeming efficient and capable. My initial thought was one of curiosity about her strong defence mechanisms which meant that although she was often in deep psychological pain, she would laugh and smile throughout our sessions together. After a few sessions I found this almost unbearable to witness and realised that my countertransference was of dread when she laughed and smiled in this way.

In supervision, I realised that I was feeling her dread, and it was all-consuming, with a sense that something catastrophic would happen. Part of her defence mechanism was to wear a mask of OK-ness, trying to convince me, and everyone else, that life was good, when it was not. As the work progressed, I discovered that being 'missed' was her story from infancy. This being missed was something I needed to keep in mind throughout our work together, as missing Camilla would have been easy: missing her real emotions and assuming she was OK; missing her emotional dysregulation and her need to be calmed and soothed, which she hid well; missing her need for constancy in her life, which she felt she had never had; missing her trauma.

In our initial sessions she found it almost impossible to put Ernest down and spent a great deal of time rocking, soothing or breastfeeding, even when her son was sound asleep. It was clear that soothing Ernest was really important to her and I wondered about co-regulation, if this soothed both of them. Even though she tried hard to hide it, I knew that Camilla was dysregulated the majority of the time, so our work together needed to begin with me providing a calm and soothing presence, to attune to her, to help her to begin to learn how to soothe herself, and to focus on our therapeutic alliance, so that we could then work with attachment.

Camilla would not leave Ernest alone for a moment, even with her husband. She refused to trust Ernest's safety with anyone and did not even trust his safety with herself. Our work was about reducing Camilla's distress around Ernest and helping her to put him down without fear, as well as to explore why she felt this way. We began by exploring what it would be like to put him down, to still touch him, but not necessarily hold him in her arms. After a few weeks she was able to bring Ernest into the room already in his car seat, and would then leave him there safely to sleep, which he often did.

Camilla was not only scared that harm would befall Ernest, but that she would in some way 'damage' her son. I could see how she struggled with intense self-doubt and anxiety. She was highly self-critical, saying she should instinctively know how to parent Ernest, and seemed to think there was something wrong because she didn't know. This was something we spent many months exploring, the 'should know', yet 'not knowing' aspect of mothering. Our work became about accessing her intuitive side, helping her to realise that she could not always 'know' and learning to tolerate this. Camilla told me that her mother expected her to know how to parent her brother, even when she was small. It was clear that her need to 'know' before she actually did came from her mother's judgment of her as the older sibling with a younger brother who she would often take care of.

Quite early on we explored Camilla's childhood, and it became instantly apparent that she had not been mothered herself. This was partly the gap in knowledge about mothering, but was also a gap in co-regulation. Camilla said her mother's life was consumed with severe mental illness, beginning with postpartum psychosis when Camilla was two, when her younger brother was born. This culminated in her mother being sectioned, and Camilla and her brother went to live with their grandparents. When her mother had another baby some years later, she experienced postpartum psychosis again. So, it was interesting that Camilla had little recollection of her childhood before the age of eight. Even as a teenager, she told me she spent more time at her grandparents than at home. This was her safe haven and her grandma was her 'rock'. Camilla did not actually know how long her mum stayed in psychiatric care, but she said it was years, not months. It was clear that this lack of mothering had impacted her a great deal.

One key point in therapy at this time was to hear my permission to parent Ernest in the way she instinctively wanted to. Camilla often asked me what

I thought about Ernest's behaviour. I would respond by gently asking her what she thought, as it was important to avoid colluding by giving advice about parenting, yet I wanted to praise her thinking. In the beginning this was like a rupture in our relationship, as Camilla found it very difficult not to be told either what to do, or what to think. Over time and with my encouragement, she was able to see that she knew much more than she thought she did about how Ernest was behaving and whether he was well or not. She would often relate to me how surprised she was that he would cry in different ways for different things. I wondered with her whether this was the beginning of Ernest being able to ask for what he wanted, with her responding accordingly. Camilla seems almost confused that Ernest might ask for what he wanted. This was completely out of her awareness, as for her, she had never even contemplated being able to do this. She described her parents as both being consumed with themselves, and totally uninterested by Camilla and her siblings.

One of the things that I enjoyed most in our work together, at this time, was helping Camilla see how Ernest watched her and responded to her, mimicking the way she moved her mouth and how he used nonverbal cues, his arms, legs and whole body sometimes, to let her know how he was emotionally, and what he needed from her and her delight and excitement at him. It was really satisfying to see how our work on enhancing our connection was filtering into and enhancing her relational connection with Ernest.

A second turning point happened when Camilla had a huge argument with her husband. He wanted Ernest to attend nursery two or three times a week to give her a break. She was distressed and horrified, as for her this was impossible to consider. I asked when it would be OK for Ernest to stay at home, so she could come to therapy without him. She replied that she did not know. Even though it was helpful for her to bring him, he was becoming more and more mobile and distracted both of us with his antics in my therapy room.

A few weeks later Camilla turned up one day alone and announced she had allowed her husband to look after Ernest for the hour of our therapy. I was pleased as I had really hoped she would begin to see the value of focusing totally on herself. When I asked her about this she said it had been important for her not to be pushed, and that she valued me leaving her to make up her own mind. This helped both of us see the extent her own self-agency was important to her and that it was beginning to develop and flourish and opened up dialogue about her leaving him on a weekly basis. Although it was clear she did have reservations, I gently encouraged her to explore with me how realistic these reservations were. At first the thought of leaving Ernest for several hours was emotionally difficult. She said it brought back feelings of terror that something would happen to him. Realising it was understandable for her to feel emotionally charged was part of helping her to understand and manage her own emotions; it was a part of her being able to differentiate between something truly catastrophic, and something that caused her a manageable level of distress. Shortly after this, she decided therapy would benefit from the lack of distraction with him being in the room. My sense was that

Camilla knew intuitively that it was time to leave Ernest for short periods of time. It had taken some time, but through intuition and our explorations, Camilla began to realise that she knew, better than anyone, how to cope with her son. Ernest never came again, although he was always metaphorically in the room with us as she talked about him a great deal.

Letting go was a theme all the way through our therapeutic relationship and the work eventually became about her ability to let go of me, as I had clearly become the good enough (m)'other' to her. We explored the term 'good enough' and whether Camilla was a 'good enough' mother. This was not easy because her father and siblings, as well as her in-laws, kept insisting Camilla was 'doing it wrong', saying that Ernest needed to be put in a cot, left to cry and that he was becoming a burden. There was also a sense of blaming Camilla for this, that she made Ernest needy. The words 'clingy' and 'a rod for your own back' were responses she received often about Ernest and Camilla's mothering style, from family members. These comments she found overwhelming and destructive to her fragile sense of self.

One day Camilla brought some old photographs of herself and her siblings from their childhood. When we talked about a picture of her, Camilla was quiet and pensive and then said she felt she was a very unhappy child. Certainly, in the photo she was not smiling and looked very uncomfortable. A few days later, she phoned me almost incoherently, sobbing with fear and grief. She arrived shortly afterwards still extremely distressed not knowing if she was coming or going, and really scared that she was experiencing psychosis. What she was experiencing was inconsolable grief, for herself, for her lost childhood, for that little girl that needed to be the mother to her brother, for the confusion and fear she felt without her own mother figure. Within the grief was extreme anger for being abandoned by her mother in such an aggressive way. She was furious with her mother for having two more children even though she was so unwell with each of them. She was also extremely angry and hurt that her mother had chosen to end her life. We explored this at length, as Camilla felt that it was the most hurtful thing her mother could have ever done when she was so close to giving birth to her first baby. The pain of her loss was huge. She said it was unbearable. She also began a process of continually questioning why this had happened. My role was to psychologically hold her in her grief, and to help her to tolerate this unbearable loss as well as to help her explore and come to terms with the impact her childhood had on her as an adult.

The focus then switched from being intensely about her mother's absence to that of her father's. One day, almost out of the blue Camilla asked me in such an angry and hurt voice, *'where was my dad?'*. She said her father had been absent nearly all the time. She described her father as 'a child' narrating several instances when her father took her and her siblings into situations that were risky and would then laugh at their fear. She said that in these instances she always told her siblings they were having a great time. Yet Camilla looked directly at me and said, *'we were terrified, and I was so angry that he behaved the way he did, laughing at us as if we were silly to be frightened'*. She was so angry and hurt by her father and the fact that he had not protected her and her siblings. She was completely unable to fathom why he had not looked after them when her mother was so ill. However, what she was most angry about was that he and her mother had conceived a third child, even when they knew she would almost certainly again have psychosis. This negatively altered her relationship with her father. They had a rupture in relationship which Camilla felt was irreparable even at the end of therapy. She was ambivalent towards him, much in the same way that he had been ambivalent towards her and she said she no longer wanted him in her life.

Another key moment was when I reflected to Camilla a similarity in relationship between herself and her husband and between her mother and herself. This opened up a dialogue about relationships and shifted her marital relationship from one of distance to one of intimacy. It was clear that Camilla had yearned to be attached to her mother, yet her mother was distant from her and kept Camilla at a distance, unless she needed something from her. Camilla also yearned to be attached to her husband, yet she would keep Ernest in the room with her and distance herself from her husband, almost using Ernest as a wedge between them. Camilla had not realised this was happening and, at first, found this realisation difficult to digest. However, with time she became more able to explore her relationship with her husband, and how she might let him close to her. Unconsciously she was terrified of him being close, as in her mind he would then abandon her, either by leaving her for another woman, by walking away, or indeed by dying. It was helpful for us to explore this level of catastrophising. She began to understand how her yearning for her mother when she was a small child, and how the message to not be close was impacting her behaviour in two different ways, with her clinging to Ernest, and with her fearing abandonment from her husband. During her therapy although she always came across to me as a terrified child, she also had an intense need to be the adult in any relationship, even with her husband. I believe this was because no one else in her family was adult enough to take responsibility for Camilla and her siblings when they were children. In particular, when she talked about her dad, I got a sense of a man who was unable to take responsibility, who felt that life was always a joke, no matter what was going on, and the severity of the situation. This sense of need to be the responsible one continued. She was the one who would visit her mother, when her siblings found it too difficult to do so. She was the one who found her mother after her mother had died. She organised the police, the funeral and all her mother's affairs afterwards even though she was by then quite heavily pregnant. Unsurprisingly, Camilla really struggled to ask for help from anyone, including me. It took her 2 years to really trust me enough to see the distraught and terrified little child inside her, although I always knew she was there.

When Camilla's therapy ended, we were both profoundly changed by the experience. Camilla was more closely connected to her husband, and her relationship with Ernest was less engulfing and more natural. She was able to tolerate uncertainty and not knowing, although she joked in our last session that she may always have the need to know. She also had the ability to regulate herself and knew that her emotions would pass. She had another baby a few years later, and although we had a few sessions together, she finally told me that she was OK; in fact she said: '*I've got this now*'. I had known from the outset that if Camilla could stay in therapy for the long term that we would be able to change her emotive responses to most things. I felt immensely proud of all she had achieved when we ended, and how able she was to cope with pretty much anything that she faced.

I learned a lot from Camilla. I already knew about the importance of the emotional bond between mother and infant. Through our work together I came to more fully understand the importance of the emotional bond and affect regulation between therapist and client and the need to calm the distress first and foremost before we can address anything else. I also experienced the opportunity which can arise through rupture and repair in the therapeutic relationship; how inevitable it is, as well as just how vital the repair is. It is from my work with her that I have gone on to research and explore affect regulation and right brain psychotherapy. Often we read about these things, but it is the experience of being with a client and doing this together that is so profound.

References

Dreyfus, H., and Dreyfus, S.E. (1986). *Mind Over Machine: The Power of Human Intuitive Expertise in the Era of the Computer.* New York: Free Press.

Fonagy, P., Gergely, G., Jurist, E.L., and Targe, M. (2004). *Affect Regulation, Mentalization, and the Development of the Self.* New York: Other Press.

Horvath, A.O., and Symonds, B.D. (1991). Relation between working alliance and outcome in psychotherapy: A meta-analysis. *Journal of Counseling Psychology*, 38, p. 139–149. https://doi.org/10.1037/0022-0167.38.2.139

Lyons-Ruth, K. (1998). Implicit relational knowing: Its role in development and psychoanalytic treatment. *Infant Mental Health Journal*, 19(3), p. 282–289.

Martin, D.J., Garske, J.P., and Davis, M.K. (2000). Relation of the therapeutic alliance with outcome and other variables: A meta-analytic review. *Journal of Consulting and Clinical Psychology*, 68, p. 438–450. PMID: 10883561.

Meares, R. (2012). *A Dissociation Model of Borderline Personality Disorder.* New York: Norton.

Muran, J.C., and Barber, J.P. (Eds) (2010). *The Therapeutic Alliance – An Evidence-Based Guide to Practice.* New York: The Guildford Press.

Ogden, T. (1982/1992). *Projective Identification and Psychotherapeutic Technique.* London: Karnac.

Paley, G., and Lawton, D. (2001). Evidence-based practice: Accounting for the importance of the therapeutic relationship in UK National Health Service provision. *Counselling and Psychotherapy Research*, 1(1), p. 12–17

Schore, A.N. (1996). The experience-dependent maturation of a regulatory system in the orbital prefrontal cortex and the origin of developmental psychopathology. *Development and Psychopathology*, 8, p. 59–87.

Schore, A.N. (2019). *The Development of the Unconscious Mind.* New York: Norton.

Spence, D. (1982). *Narrative Truth and Historical Truth: Meaning and Interpretation in Psychoanalysis.* New York: W.W. Norton & Company.

14 Using Creativity and Creative Methods in Psychotherapy

This chapter is devoted to creativity, which I use in my work when working with maternal mental illness, and in particular with postpartum psychosis. I use these techniques to unlock the silent aspects of experience and to free up new connections. This helps to counteract women's feelings of being silenced and remaining silent, due to their experiences of being on the margins of society, of feeling judged and shamed of their experiences. It also gives women another way to express their experiences. Creativity brings to the fore elements of the client's unconscious process, implicitly through the transferential domain and explicitly through the narrative form. What I have found is that often the creative element or object becomes the key that unlocks something within the unconscious, allowing it to become conscious and thus be explored co-creatively and then integrated. Creativity can also allow the silent parts of our process to have a voice in dialogue. When working with marginalised clients, this becomes particularly important as they often feel silenced or indeed silence themselves. Using creativity or a creative object as a symbol of their illness offers a voice for those unspoken parts. In this chapter, I give a brief description of what I mean by creativity, then I go on to explain some of the creative methods I use with clients. The chapter ends with a clinical vignette to show how I used a creative object with a client who had experienced postpartum psychosis and the positive impact this had in instigating change in her therapy.

Creativity enriches the practice of psychotherapy, particularly in the way it is able to unlock unconscious processes and silence and offers both therapist and client the freedom to explore and learn. As early as 1954, Carl Rogers extolled the importance of creativity in our work and its ability to bring novelty (the new) into therapy when he wrote that creativity is *'the emergence in action of a novel relational product, growing out of the uniqueness of the individual on the one hand, and the materials, events, people, or circumstances of his life on the other'* (1954, p. 251). I believe creativity enhances healing and transformation in our clients because it transcends familiarity and overcomes the discipline of words (Mead, 1995). It also allows for right brain to right brain communication which is a primary part of change in psychotherapy. For me, it is also a way to combat classifying maternal mental illness by symptoms and diagnostic categories.

DOI: 10.4324/9781003154891-16

Throughout this book, I have highlighted the importance of the specificity of maternal mental illness, that each woman will have her own unique experience and that we must not box women solely into categories or symptoms. I believe that creativity brings forth this specificity and is a way to honour her uniqueness of experience. Using creative techniques and creativity is of huge benefit to human experience and to psychotherapy, as it offers an alternative lens through which to see the 'unseeable' of the client we are working with. It also allows us the choice to step into the unknown together, moving beyond what we can see and hear. As Pat Ogden said: *'to be creative is to experiment with new ideas, concepts, activities, and actions in ways that transcend rules and habitual modes of thinking, feeling and moving'* (2018, p. 92).

What is creativity?

I use three particular words to explicate what I mean by creativity: *novelty, effectiveness* (Cropley, 2011) and *originality* (Andreasen, 2011). This chapter does not have the scope to explore creativity to its full extent, as that would be a book in its own right. However, to further clarify what I mean, I use *'characterised by flashes of insight that arise from unconscious reservoirs of the mind and brain'* (Andreasen, 2011, p. 42) as a way to illustrate what I think of as creativity. So how does creativity occur? We all have moments of flashes of insight. Ritter and Dijksterhuis call those moments in humans when the flashes of insight can occur as the 'incubation period'. Their belief is that those moments are times when we can unlock the *'unconscious foundations of the incubation period'* (2014, p. 215). For me, the incubation period might be another term for free association – the psychoanalytic technique whereby we are able to express the contents of our thoughts, with no censorship, spontaneously speaking without restricting ourselves as a way to access the unconscious. Research shows that unconscious processes play a significant part in creativity (Andreasen, 2011). I believe this is a bilateral process, that creativity can also play a significant part in unlocking the unconscious.

In psychotherapy, we are not only interested in the narrative form. We use visual cues – movements, gestures, behaviour – in a diagnostic way and interweave them into the narrative as a way to inform the process. Using these more visual forms brings in immediacy and authenticity (Spencer, 2011). Creativity, both visual and imaginary, brings a new experience. The new experience is part of the change process in psychotherapy (Marks-Tarlow, 2018), and brings new responses, new narrative that highlights the change. For example, when a client is stuck, they may tell the same story many times over. This allows me to know that not only are they stuck, but that the therapy may also be stuck. Perhaps the client has not processed what they need to and what they are showing me is that their process has not yet begun to shift and change. This gives me valuable insight into their process and offers me an opportunity to bring in something new to unstick the process and a possibility for using a creative technique. I will know we are both freer when the narrative begins to slowly shift and change.

Creativity is helpful in two different ways – explicitly and implicitly. It can unlock silence and bring elements of the unconscious to the fore so these can be explored together, explicitly using the narrative and implicitly using the transferential domain. Natasha Mauthner, in her research on narratives of postpartum depression talks about how women silence themselves: '*women … describe losing their own voices to those of others – healthcare professionals, family members, and friends – telling them how they should think and feel, and behave as mothers. Although they question these voices [...] they nevertheless feel under pressure and compelled to conform to them*'. Using a creative object as a tool to explore the silent aspects of experience can offer a voice for the silence. The object seems to speak of itself (Haynes, 2022). Within the transferential domain, we can explore what Cornell and Landaiche call '*implicit memory of primary relational patterns*' (2006, p. 203). These primary relational patterns are those patterns laid down in the first 2 years of childhood when our brain is undergoing huge developmental processes. These are the processes that are the foundation of every other aspect of our life, interpersonally and intrapsychically and so exploring them is vital, particularly with clients with early developmental trauma.

Using creative methods

There are many different types of creative methods used in therapy – sand trays, art therapy, picture cards, and creative writing, for example. What we choose to use does not matter, it is more of personal choice. I use several alternative creative methods of my own with my clients. Often, I will invite a client to bring in an object, anything they choose, for us to explore together as a representation of their experience. The idea is for the visual to complement the narrative and for it to become part of the psychotherapeutic process. I am also interested in silence as I find it is an underutilised resource in therapy. A client can remain silent for many different reasons – the somatic child (a TA term to describe a very young internal, preverbal part of self where experiences and disturbances are felt only at a bodily level) may be unable to narrate their experience, the silence may be filled with the unspoken or the unspeakable. Silence can be privileged, cultural and powerful, and creative methods can offer a voice for the silent aspects through the dialogue generated between therapist and client. Women's silence is often cultural – women talk about silence being a part of their culture, and Dana Jack and Alisha Ali edited an entire book called Silencing the Self Across Cultures (2010) dedicated to giving new psychological and social perspectives on women's depression from across the world.

Verb sequencing, reverie, intuition, symbols and metaphors are other creative techniques I use. Intuition is fed by those tiny implicit cues such as paralinguistics – prosody, pitch, volume, intonation or the visual, facial and postural cues that come from the right brain processes formed in the first 2 years of life. These cues are part of what Lyons-Ruth calls implicit relational knowing (1998). These implicit cues help to guide my intuition about what is happening within a client and are precious to me. They show the depth of our relationship and connection, and although we may be forming dialogue around intense negative emotional experiences, these intuitive absorptions allow me to know I am fully tuned into my client, much like a mother can know that she is fully attuned to her infant. These implicit cues were shaped in my client a long time before her cognitive and verbal abilities which developed later in childhood. Implicit cues are much faster than explicit cognitive ones (thinking, analysing, deciding, acting upon) and are part of what Beatrice Beebe documents as those moments so important upon the future attachment of infant and parent, those tiny moments of discordance or synchrony (Beebe et al., 2010, 2012) which Tronick et al. first showed us in his influential video – The Still Face Experiment (1975).

Marks-Tarlow shows us how intuition is vibrant and alive in therapy:

> *Where theory is static, intuition is alive. Where theory exists outside of real time, intuition involves immersion within lived moments. When clinicians become immersed in this fashion, we often attain states of flow (Csíkszentmihályi, 1990, 1996) with our patients. When in a state of flow, therapists get caught up in the throes of implicit processes as intuitively guided.*
>
> (Marks-Tarlow, 2018)

She goes on to explain that this is the realm of intersubjectivity – a place of entwinement of the self and other both physiologically and psychologically (2008). This is a place of two-person psychotherapy (Stark, 1999) – a place of attunement in which a client's defence mechanisms can be safely explored and released, unlocking, in turn, the client's own intuitive processes in their right brain.

Temporal sequencing of verbs is helpful in showing us where the client is in their process. In the first sessions, I notice that the clients, when talking about past trauma, for example, talk about it in the present tense, allowing me to know that the trauma is not over for them and that they seem unable to update their contextual representation of the traumatic event and may have general context-processing difficulties. As treatment progresses, I then notice that the tense they are speaking in can begin to change. When they relate their negative experiences, it may finally be in the past tense, showing movement and change in process. Again, these may seem almost imperceptible to therapists. However, I have found that tuning into these clues is a useful way for me to mark our progress together.

Reverie is also a client process which benefits from gentle creative exploration. I find that the creative object the client brings can often bring with it reverie. What I mean by this is it is almost as if they are re-experiencing something from the past, as if caught in a daydream, or a place of silent musing, causing them to lose connection with us and to seem to be in a haze. Paying careful attention to these moments and recognising them can help the client to see how often they are disconnecting with us, it gives us behavioural clues about dissociation and the level of trauma they are experiencing. I am really tuned into my countertransference when my client is in reverie. This offers another way of being responsive to the unconscious phenomena which are at play and offers a way to help us understand our clients experience through somatisation. However, clients do not always respond to our offerings of these transferential experiences. If they do not, then it is prudent to let go of them.

Flashes of insight may come as visual metaphors, music, hunches, words or emergent symbols. These flashes originate in the implicit realm and are often of a sensory nature (we feel them in our body, perhaps), and are emotional. These can be such useful ways to help our clients make meaning of their experience and can guide us intuitively in the pathway to take with a client. Metaphors the client uses are helpful, and Daniel Stern talks about the key challenge in psychotherapy as the importance of finding the central metaphor (1985). When metaphors also begin to shift and change, again this is information on the process of change.

In order to show one way of how I use creativity, I have included a clinical vignette below, which describes how I used my client Laura's creative object to unstick her process. Laura came to me a few months after she had been discharged from her local MBU. This vignette will be published as part of an article called 'Using creative methods to research TA psychotherapy' in the Transactional Analysis Journal. It is reprinted here with the kind permission of the editor. The article was originally written for Transactional Analysts. To enable it to be more readable to a wider audience, I have removed the TA terms and put them in an easily understandable format.

Client vignette

Laura

Laura came to see me 2 months after experiencing postpartum psychosis. She was terrified she would have psychosis again and could not make sense of why this had happened to her. It was clear she was completely traumatised by her experience of psychosis. My first focus was to alleviate her distress and support her frightened inner child so that we could begin to unravel what had happened. It became apparent early on that her ability to affect-regulate was limited and she was reliant on others to calm and reassure her.

A few months into therapy, I asked Laura to bring an object to our next session together that represented her therapy so far because Laura could not see a change in herself. Yet I could see she had changed a great deal. Her inner child was, in her mind, hampering her ability to *'get up and get on'* with her life. She dismissed her inner child and instead had very negative thoughts, castigating herself so thoroughly and painfully. She also negated the trauma she had experienced, berating herself for not '*being over it*', which I found painful but necessary to witness. I needed to know her intrapsychic process so that I could help her understand the part her terrified child played for her. She also unconsciously needed me to witness that part, to understand the way this part of her literally stopped her from getting out of bed and looking after her baby. She related watching her husband care for their daughter from across the room, feeling detached and miserable, totally unable to move towards them and re-connect with them both, completely stuck in passivity. I knew I needed to help her connect with her somatic child so that she might then re-connect with her husband and connect and bond with her baby.

The object Laura chose was a pencil case. The case was black with colourful flowers appliquéd on top. At first, she said the pencil case was necessary so she could '*zip*' her psychosis away, so she no longer had it anymore. I realised that this was a parallel to her own process. She wanted to 'zip' her inner child away, shut her down, shut her up and no longer feel her anymore. In her mind, this would free her to get on with her life, to get herself out of her bed, to '*get up and get back to work*', something she kept saying she needed to do. Zipping her psychosis away meant she would be safe from it, tucked away where it could not escape. This sense of the psychosis being separate, a thing that had attacked her, is something I often hear from women who have recently experienced it. Helping Laura to understand that the psychosis was her, a symptom of her extreme distress and internal to her, not separate from and therefore out of her control, was a large part of our work together.

The colour of the pencil case – black – was emblematic of her experience after psychosis, the black hole she felt she was in at that moment, unable to engage with anyone and completely incapable (in her mind) of looking after her baby. Yet, when I noticed the colourful flowers on the outside with her, her narrative began to change. She began to talk about the flowers as a sense of hope for her, therapy was her hope. I wondered if she felt the flowers could cover up the black, the dark hole. I also spoke of the black offering a juxtaposition to the colourful flowers and gently was curious whether this might be a part of her therapy, the dark and the light (colour). We talked about how the colour of the flowers was enhanced with the black background and I wondered with Laura if her psychosis and the knowledge of herself it was bringing was similar.

We explored her inner child, slowly helping Laura gain an understanding of her past history and how this had played a significant part in her psychosis. The past was something Laura had also zipped away, unable to go back there for fear of what she might find, constantly running away from it. Laura began to realise she was doing the same with her psychosis, running towards work so she would no longer have to face her lack of connection with her baby and her lost connection with her husband. She began to grieve her loss, which was a significant turning point. She began to understand almost imperceptibly how important and yet damaged her inner child was. She grieved the lack in her childhood, her need to always be the parent for herself and her sister, to be the sensible one to step up and take care of them both. Her mother was always away at work, and her father was 'away in his head', struggling with severe mental illness.

Another turning point was when Laura began to understand her fear. As a child, she said she was always scared walking home from school, of what she might find, that today might be the day her father had finally committed suicide, something she is still scared of now, 30 years later. She talked about having felt terrified for the whole of her life. We explored the part her husband played in making her feel safe, he is a police officer.

Towards the end of her therapy, I spoke about the significance of her pencil case and how it had unlocked so much for us. Laura laughed and said how ironic it was that she chose something to 'zip' away when in actual fact, it had 'unzipped' her understanding. For Laura, the flowers became a metaphor for positivity over the blackness. She also decided to 'empty' her case of the psychosis and instead fill it with the metaphorical 'tools' she said she had learnt during therapy. Tools to help her if she had a bad day and found getting out of bed a struggle. In actuality, she did not need those tools, although I imagine the pencil case will always hold special meaning. Laura chose not to go back to work for another 6 months. She began to engage and connect with her daughter, even finding that she had the capacity to play, something she was scared of. Playing had not featured in her childhood at all.

References

Andreasen, N. (2011) A journey into chaos: Creativity and the unconscious. *Mens Sana Monographs*, 9(1), p. 42–53. https://doi.org/10.4103/0973-1229.77424

Beebe, B., Jaffe, J., Markese, S., Buck, K., Chen, H., Cohen, P., Bahrick, L., Andres, H., and Feldstein, S. (2010). The origins of 12-month attachment: A microanalysis of 4-month mother-infant interaction. *Attachment & Human Development*, 12(1–2), p. 3–141. https://doi.org/10.1080/14616730903338985

Beebe, B., Lachmann, F., Markese, S., and Bahrick, L. (2012). On the origins of disorganized attachment and internal working models: Paper I. A dyadic systems approach. *Psychoanalytic Dialogues*, 22(2), p. 253–272. https://doi.org/10.1080/10481885.2012.666147

Cornell, W.F., and Landaiche, N.M. III. (2006) Impasse and intimacy: Applying Berne's concept of script protocol. *Transactional Analysis Journal*, 36(3), p. 196–213. https://doi.org/10.1177/036215370603600304

Cropley, A.J. (2011). Definitions of creativity. In M.A. Runco & S.R. Pritzker (Eds), *Encyclopedia of Creativity*. pp. 511–524. San Diego, CA: Academic Press.

Csíkszentmihályi, M. (1990). *Flow: The Psychology of Optimal Experience*. New York: Harper & Row.

Csíkszentmihályi, M. (1996). *Creativity: Flow and the Psychology of Discovery and Invention*. New York: Harper Collins.

Haynes, E. (2022). Bridging the gap between research and practice: Using creative methods to research transactional analysis psychotherapy. *Transactional Analysis Journal*, 52(1). https://doi.org/10.1080/03621357.2022.2019406

Jack, D.C., and Ali, A. (2010). *Silencing the Self across Cultures – Depression and Gender in the Social World*. New York: Oxford University Press.

Lyons-Ruth, K. (1998). Implicit relational knowing: It's role in development and psychoanalytic treatment. *Infant Mental Health Journal*, 19(3), p. 282–289. CCC 0163-9641/98/030282-08

Marks-Tarlow, T. (2018). Awakening clinical intuition: Creativity and play. In T. Marks-Tarlow, M. Solomon & D.J. Siegel (Eds), *Play & Creativity in Psychotherapy*. New York: W.W. Norton & Company.

Mead, M. (1995). Visual anthropology in a discipline of worlds. In P. Hocking (Ed.), *Principles of Visual Anthropology*. pp 3–10. Berlin: Mouton de Gruyter.

Ogden, P. (2018). Play, creativity, and movement vocabulary. In T. Marks-Tarlow, M. Solomon & D.J. Siegel (Eds), *Play & Creativity in Psychotherapy*. New York: W.W. Norton & Company.

Ritter, S.M., and Dijksterhuis, A. (2014). Creativity – The unconscious foundations of the incubation period. *Frontiers of Human Neuroscience*, 8, p. 215. https://doi.org/10.3389/fnhum.2014.00215

Rogers, C. (1954). Toward a theory of creativity. *A Review of General Semantics*, 11(4), p. 249–260.

Spencer, S. (2011). *Visual Research Methods in the Social Science: Awakening Visions*. London: Routledge.

Stark, M. (1999). *Modes of Therapeutic Action*. Northvale, NJ: Jason Aronson Inc.

Stern, D.N. (1985). *The Interpersonal World of the Infant: A View from Psychoanalysis and Developmental Psychology*. New York: Basic Books.

Tronick, E., Adamson, L.B., Als, H., and Brazelton, T.B. (1975). Infant emotions in normal and pertubated interactions. Paper presented at the biennial meeting of the Society for Research in Child Development, Denver, CO.

15 Neurodivergence and Motherhood

Co-authored with Holly Radford

What actually is neurodivergence? The Cambridge English Online Dictionary (2021) defines the word neurodivergent as 'having or related to a type of brain that is often considered as different from what is usual, for example that of someone who has autism'. Neurodivergence is extremely important to highlight within this book because the most recent research shows that psychotherapists lack knowledge of neurodiversity and in particular their knowledge and self-perceived competency to diagnose and treat autistic patients was lower than with all other diagnoses (Lipinski et al., 2021). I therefore wanted to include this chapter to help psychotherapists working with a client who is neurodivergent. Many women who have mental health conditions may also be autistic and may or may not have a formal diagnosis or awareness. Therefore, the likelihood that psychotherapists will see someone with maternal mental illness who is also neurodivergent is high. This lack of knowledge is a reported barrier for treatment for women with autism (Lipinski et al., 2021). I cannot cover every aspect of neurodivergence in this chapter, so I have chosen to concentrate on autism and attention-deficit hyperactivity disorder (ADHD), as these are the most prevalent.

I will begin by briefly describing neurodiversity/neurodivergence, then describe autism and ADHD, including their prevalence. To counteract the lack of knowledge, I will highlight elements which are important for psychotherapists to know about autism and motherhood. I have also included some of the narratives we might hear, such as:

- What it is like to be a neurodivergent parent
- What it is like to be a neurodivergent parent, with a neurodivergent child
- What it is like to be a neurodivergent parent, with a neurotypical child
- What it is like to be a neurotypical parent, but with a neurodivergent child

I end the chapter with some things to think about when working with a neurodivergent client. My hope is that we, as professionals, can gain some understanding of the difficulties that might occur for these women and parents

DOI: 10.4324/9781003154891-17

and give us more clarity on how this might impact their psychotherapy so that we can enable and enhance their therapeutic process.

Semantics

First, it is important to be clear about terminology, as this is often an area of confusion. Neurodiversity refers to a group of people of a range of neurotypes, including neurotypical. This term is used to talk about the range of diversity in humans. An individual, therefore, cannot be neurodiverse, as diversity is the property of a group. Psychotherapists might have a group of clients who are neurodiverse (for example, some may be neurotypical, some may be autistic, some may have ADHD). The singular term is neurodivergent and this term refers to an individual who has a neurotype that deviates from the majority or predominant neurotype. When we use the term neurodivergence/neurodivergent we mean minority neurotypes (for example, people with autism, ADHD, dyslexia, dyscalculia, dysgraphia, dyspraxia, Tourette Syndrome, OCD and epilepsy). There is also a huge range of diversity in the way that traits are experienced. Autism and Asperger's actually mean the same thing. The term autism refers to anyone with a diagnosis of autism or Asperger's, and if someone also experiences a co-occurring learning disability or language delay/impairment, this is specified separately.

Autism is not synonymous with learning disabilities nor with using non-speaking forms of communication, although these can co-occur. About half of the autistic population do not have a learning disability/intellectual impairment, and about 30% are totally or partially non-speaking and use other forms of communication (i.e. text-based communication such as emails and text, or use alternative communication devices) (Anderson et al., 2007).

Some autistic women will also have ADHD and/or other forms of neurodivergence. This may alter the way that they experience autistic traits and can have an impact on how they experience pregnancy and motherhood. For example, autistic people have a strong preference for order and routine, whilst people with ADHD have a strong drive for novelty. Autistic people can find it distressing when a routine is changed or interrupted, and both autistic people and those with ADHD can find it difficult to implement and stick to routines or organise themselves due to challenges with executive functioning. This can make routine-making in motherhood particularly difficult. In some ways it feels like autism and ADHD pull in opposite directions, which can present unique challenges when trying to parent.

Autism

Autism is a broad spectrum of neurodevelopmental differences. In the medical model it is called Autism Spectrum Disorder. However, the term autism spectrum conditions (ASC) is now a preferable term as it is less stigmatising (Dudas et al., 2017). Autistic people have different perceptions and experiences of the world and relate to others in ways which differ from neurotypical/non-autistic norms. These differences in social communication (APA, 2013) can cause autistic people to be misunderstood by those around them, and differences in sensory perception can be challenging when sensory needs are not accommodated. The prevalence of autism worldwide is given as around 1% of the population (Brugha et al., 2011), although most autistic adults are undiagnosed and many may be unaware that they are autistic. As with other medical tools, the diagnostic assessment tools for autism are based on males and as such are heavily biased towards men. This has caused difficulties and delay in recognising autism in women and girls (Devokut et al., 2017; Kreiser & White, 2014).

There is a medical model of autism which views autism as deficits or impairments which need to be fixed or changed by medical treatment. However, there are other models that form a counterargument that it is not the autism itself which is problematic. The human rights model is about acceptance of disability as a normal part of the variation in humans and this model validates an individual's rights. The human rights model is interested in discrimination and exclusion and how these occur through social policies and societal structures. There is also the social model which is interested in accommodating all autistic people into society.

Co-occurrence of autism and mental health difficulties is common and research from Hofvander et al. shows that more than half of adults with autism have mental health disorders (2009), with anxiety the highest. There is also co-occurrence of autism and ADHD, with around 28% being diagnosed with both (Lai et al., 2019). Of those who need mental health help, most (73%) actually ask for help (Baldwin & Costley, 2015). In maternal mental illness, it is important for psychotherapists to have a willingness and openness to treat adults on the spectrum. Lack of knowledge is reported as one of the highest predictors of a lack of willingness. Au-Yeung et al. suggest that there is an inability for psychotherapists to differentiate between mental health conditions and autism traits (2019), so knowledge can help with counteracting misconceptions and outdated beliefs. Until very recently, neurodiversity was not a part of the curriculum in psychotherapeutic training.

Two final things to consider when working with neurodivergent mothers is the high levels of suicidal ideation and the high instances of trauma. Between 30% and 50% of autistic people have considered suicide (Balfe & Tantam, 2010; Raja, 2014) and two-thirds of autistic adults have reported a lifetime experience of suicidal thoughts and one-third had planned or attempted suicide (Cassidy et al., 2014). Autistic women experience high levels of prejudice, discrimination, victimisation, bullying, harassment and abuse. One difficulty with autistic women and trauma is that a broader range of life events (for example, non-DSM-V trauma) are experienced as traumatic and therefore may result in higher levels of post-traumatic stress disorder (PTSD) (Haruvi-Lamden et al., 2020; Rumball, Happé & Grey, 2020). Autistic women are significantly more likely than autistic men to experience sexual assault (Reuben, Stanzione & Singleton, 2021). So, it is important to think about whether you are treating maternal mental illness and trauma when working with mothers who are neurodivergent.

Attention deficit hyperactivity disorder (ADHD)

According to DSM-V (APA, 2013) people with ADHD experience hyperactivity, inattention, and impulsivity, can find it difficult to screen out distractions, often have poor organisational skills, and some have difficulties with restlessness. Medication is often prescribed for ADHD, and a longitudinal study by Uchida et al. shows that stimulant use seems to be associated with more positive outcomes. Such as a reduced risk of substance use, better functional outcomes and a decreased risk of co-morbid psychiatric disorders (2018), which was corroborated by the systematic literature review by Boland et al. (2020). ADHD traits can be diagnosed in both childhood and adulthood and there are different presentations. Most people with ADHD have what is called 'inattentive' ADHD. Yet the common misconception is to think that someone with an ADHD diagnosis is physically hyperactive. In reality, hyperactivity can be mental or verbal, and some people with ADHD do not experience hyperactivity at all.

There is a tension between the medical discourse of ADHD which sees those diagnosed as having a biomedical brain disorder (Singh, 2013) and other models. The social context model emphasises the role of familial and social context in which the child grows up and is more aligned with the diagnosis being more frequently seen in children experiencing family disadvantages, such as unstable home environments, divorce, parental mental illness and the use of illicit substances within the family. However, a counterargument, similar to that in autism, would be that ADHD is a natural part of neurodiversity, and the problem is not the person with ADHD; rather it is the environment and the lack of understanding from others that is more problematic. Brinkman (2016) states that there has been an increased search for diagnoses to explain human behaviours, reactions, emotions and transitional developments. The narrative from a parent to a doctor may be 'there is something wrong with my child'; for example, the child is overeating, or considered to be talking too much or their behaviour is too much. Within the medical discourse, there is often a belief that children will 'grow out of' ADHD. However, it is now known that this is not true and that it is a lifelong diagnosis (Courchesne, Campbell & Solso, 2011).

On a worldwide basis, ADHD is the most common neurodevelopmental disorder. The rates of identification/diagnosis have increased rapidly over the last few decades (LeFever Watson et al., 2014; Visser et al., 2013). Yet, it is not clear whether the prevalence of ADHD itself has increased. The increase may be due to improved or more accurate diagnosis of autistic women and girls, for example, or of inattentive ADHD. It would appear that the prevalence of ADHD is around 3% of the adult population worldwide (Zhu et al., 2017).

Research has been completed on whether there is an impact on pregnancy, birth and early parent–child interaction from maternal ADHD (Kittel-Schneider et al., 2021). This systematic review also looked at the risks of both stimulant medication and no medication in pregnancy and during breast-feeding. The conclusion was that due to the behavioural aspects of ADHD, there might be a likelihood of unplanned and teenage pregnancies in girls and women with ADHD. However, being able to counteract this is difficult as women and girls are less likely to be diagnosed with ADHD or identified as autistic and so might not know they were at risk of unplanned pregnancies. The research found that having ADHD could have a negative impact on parent and child interaction in the early stages after birth. Amphetamines seemed to have no risk for any type of congenital malformations and little risk to placental functioning and the conclusion was that these were relatively safe to be taken in pregnancy. Methylphenidate showed a small risk for birth defects, particularly cardiovascular, as well as impacts on placental functioning and there was evidence of perinatal complications, although Kittel-Schneider et al. did report that there was a lack of clarity as to whether this was due to the maternal ADHD or the medication. Some studies they reviewed showed that exposure to ADHD medication was associated with higher rates of admission to neonatal intensive care units (Nörby, Winbladh & Källén, 2017). Poulton and team researched the association between ADHD medication and neonatal resuscitation, neonatal admission and an increase in C-sections, finding these risks increased when the woman was taking the medication (2018). Kittel-Schneider and team also found that parents with a child with autism or an ADHD diagnosis were generally more stressed.

Understanding autism and ADHD in mothers and parents

In order to counteract some of the lack of knowledge in psychotherapists, I thought it would be helpful to offer some guidance for working with autism/ADHD and motherhood. We all hold unconscious bias and make assumptions, so this section is to try and help offset these.

Autistic mothers/birth parents may have very different experiences of pregnancy, birth and the post-natal period. They are at increased risk of a pre-term birth because of higher levels of stress (Behrman & Butler, 2007). Sensory differences can make pregnancy and birth challenging (Ben-Sasson et al., 2009; Keuler et al., 2011), as autistic people can be hyper-sensitive to sensory stimuli. These can include touch (for example, clinicians touching them, breastfeeding support, partners touching them and breastfeeding their baby); sound (hospital sounds, baby crying, noisy baby toys, noise levels at baby groups and health clinics); interoception (feelings inside the body such as changes during pregnancy, birth, post-natal changes, nausea, hunger), all of which can be overwhelming, painful, and distressing. This can make it difficult to adapt to motherhood (Sundeline et al., 2018) and mothers can feel overwhelmed, isolated and misunderstood. Many autistic women/birth parents find this sensory aspect the hardest part of being a parent. Difficulties include feeling the baby moving inside, which can feel unbearable. The perception from autistic mothers may be that other non-autistic mothers do not ever feel this sensory overload, although I do hear narratives of fear in pregnancy that the baby is 'an alien' or some non-human life form rather than a real baby from many mothers, not just autistic ones. Birth, in particular, can feel like a sensory overload, and for some being touched by medical professionals was 'horrific'. However, these types of sensory overloads do not finish with birth. A sense of feeling invaded bodily, both by the medical profession but also by the infant, whilst breastfeeding, and if the infant constantly climbs on her and needs to be rocked and cuddled, can make some mothers struggle with every-day parenting. Others felt as if their skin was unable to tolerate more touch (Talcer, Duffy & Pedlow, 2021).

The double empathy problem (Milton, 2012) may be highlighted in ther-apy and is really important to understand. Non-autistic people find it hard to relate to, understand and empathise with autistic people's experiences and find it hard to interpret their behaviour and mental states, which can lead to misunderstandings in interactions between autistic and non-autistic people.

Many parenting, communication and relationship expectations are based upon normative assumptions which may not apply to autistic people. This is an area where we may need to be particularly vigilant to unconscious bias in therapy. It can be useful to explore any differences we perceive in supervi-sion. Autistic parents may parent differently, may relate to others and com-municate differently and may have different priorities for, and experiences of, relationships. An autistic parent's relationship with their autistic child may look and sound very different from the relationship between a non-autistic parent and their non-autistic child.

Autistic women and parents may relate to and experience emotions differently. They may not use typical emotion words as they may find it hard to identify emotions and express them (alexithymia) (Bird & Cook, 2013), but this does not mean they don't experience them. Often, autistic parents will have a heightened awareness of their own and others' emotional states, and this intense empathy can cause hyper-arousal and be overwhelming. Also, emotions and feelings may manifest in physical sensations. Anxiety, for example, is often felt physically and is a response to the environment (sensory triggers) rather than a response to cognitive thoughts or worries (Top et al., 2019).

Autistic parents may have difficulties maintaining friendships and social relationships during times of transition and change, such as during pregnancy or postnatally. Again, they feel that other parents don't seem to have the same experiences or challenges, so they can't relate to them or understand their experiences. Autistic parents are more likely to struggle going out to meet other parents and socialise because they are already exhausted from the overwhelming sensory experience of being a parent and need more quiet time on their own to recover. They may need to carefully balance social time with rest and recovery at home.

Narratives of neurodiversity

Being a neurodivergent mother with a neurodivergent child

Research into the narratives of autistic mothers is limited. However, Dugdale et al. have researched this by exploring the narratives of nine women, seven of whom were autistic mothers with autistic children. They discovered that sharing diagnosis with their child can help mothers to feel closer to their child, sharing *'a special bond'*, *'common ground to bond with and talk about'*, or *'being peas in a pod'* (2021). This sharing of diagnosis can lead to parenting challenges, with a sense that the parent therefore understands the child better, and thus may be expected to do the majority of the child-rearing by the neurotypical parent. They also found that the mothers they interviewed felt a need for routine, as this helped with consistency for their children. However, some found it really difficult to do routines and spoke of them as being like *'demand overload'*.

It is quite possible that autistic mothers may feel misunderstood, judged or discounted by others, and can be perceived as coping well when they actually are not. Stigma was reported in the research by Dugdale et al., with some mothers feeling significantly dismissed when voicing concerns about their children. This seemed to be around a lack of understanding of autism and a need for training of medical professionals. However, the participants in the study all felt an intense connection with their children, which could feel overwhelming at times but on the whole was positive: *'Despite the challenges of motherhood, the shared experience between mothers and their children in this study highlighted a narrative of enduring connection and love'* (Dugdale et al., 2021, p. 1982).

Having an autistic child when you are neurotypical

What does it mean to discover your child is autistic or is on the autism spectrum, when you or your partner are not? This can be a difficult challenge, which can change a woman's outlook on life and rock her sense of identity (Emerson, 2003). It can also place huge strain on the family and increase difficulties in parenting and family relationships (Wieland et al., 2014). For some women there was a need to change their idealized image of their child from a 'healthy' to 'disordered' child, and all that might entail (Harwood, McLean & Durkin, 2007). Other aspects, which could be seen as the strain an autistic child placed on families, were the tensions with partners, and siblings; a sense of helplessness and frustration, of not knowing what to do, and of fear of their child's future; as well as stigma, and a sense that social possibilities were in decline (Papadopoulos, 2021). Some women expressed a lack of knowledge about how to manage their child's difficulties (Lin, 2010). And there is evidence to show that mothers are impacted by the behaviour of their neurodivergent child, as they are more likely to experience PTSD (Roberts et al., 2014).

Having ADHD and being a mother – Distraction

This last section includes narrative from Natalie, a mother with ADHD who agreed to be interviewed in April 2021for this chapter. One of the difficulties in working with ADHD is the difficulty with the client 'disappearing' due to distraction. This is important to know for psychotherapy and this happened with Natalie in our interview together. This can have a sense of 'derailing' the process and needs to be thought through for the benefit of the therapeutic process.

Shame, guilt and fear seem to be emotions that many mothers, and particularly mothers with ADHD and autism, can feel and certainly Natalie felt this strongly:

> *The key things that have affected my mothering of my children are a deep feeling of shame, of guilt and fear, as well as moments of anger. So generally speaking, very intense emotions, much more intense than the situation calls for. The shame is about not knowing anything that I feel every mother knows, the shame of needing help and not having anyone to rely on and the shame for not coping, for losing my temper, for becoming depressed and exhausted.*

Another element expressed by Natalie is the difficulty with intense emotions and sometimes not being able to express these emotions in a fruitful way. Women with autism may find it hard to identify emotions and express them, but often can have intense emotional states which can be overwhelming. Others have been taught from a young age that their experiences and feelings are incorrect, wrong, or invalid (*'It's not too hot'*, *'it's not too bright'*, *'you're fine'*, *'there is nothing wrong with you'*, *'if you cry I'll be cross and I'll take your toy away'*). The messages they have received, often from an early age, are that their feelings don't matter, they are not real and that other people's needs supersede how they are feeling. In this way, they learn to switch off and disengage from their feelings, leading to an inability to feel, or their feelings can manifest in explosive outbursts

> *When Clara was very young and I was feeding her in her high-chair, if she threw food on the floor, a very normal behaviour for a young child, I would get into a hardly controllable rage, like a pressure cooker. I felt so guilty each time I did that. I think I did it because I did not have the words to express my anger in a grounded and healthy way.*

Another element that Natalie highlights is how difficult it can be for women with autism or ADHD to trust people. Although she said that how she experienced this was contradictory:

> *I find it hard to trust when people are kind to me and then I trust complete strangers without questioning anything… I seem to make the same mistakes of trusting people too fast. It seems that I want to include and trust everyone at the expense of myself or my own family.*

> [This has caused me to] *have failed to protect my children and I have made myself ill with obsessive thoughts about how I failed them. The worst thing was that I was left with my obsessions. I almost became mad because of this.*

Natalie is a great mother and has a very close bond with her children. Being a neurodivergent mother has not negatively impacted her children at all. In fact, quite the opposite, what it has done is give the children the ability to attune to, be compassionate and empathise with children who are struggling and who may be neurodivergent.

This chapter can only be brief. However, the aim is to highlight neurodivergency and its prevalence. To conclude, a neurodivergent client has shared with me her thoughts on helpful tips for psychotherapists. These may be things we already know, but are useful reminders about those elements that we may take for granted with all our clients. Yet, some of them can help to reduce distress in a new client who may be neurodivergent.

Things to think about as a psychotherapist working with a neurodivergent client

Be clear with your client, say what you mean, and mean what you say. Autistic people tend to be very direct and honest in their communication and will not read between the lines, interpreting your words as being exactly what you mean.

Autism challenges executive functioning. It is important to ask what your client's communication preferences are. For some, phone calls are distressing, so they might prefer text messages or emails. Some autistic people prefer zoom appointments rather than face-to-face. However, others find zoom difficult and prefer being in the room together. It is important not to be rigid in your offer of therapy. For clarity, consider sending reminders about appointments, and written confirmation of any appointments made.

Autistic people can find uncertainty and unpredictability anxiety-inducing, particularly if they don't know exactly what is expected of them in sessions, or what your expectations are. It is useful to make this as concrete and explicit as possible. Consider discussing what might happen in the next session – whether they would like to continue talking about something, bring something new, or whether it is easier for them for you to propose something. Prior to the next session they might feel the need to send you an agenda of things they would like to talk about to reduce uncertainty and unpredictability. For similar reasons, on your website you could have a photo of yourself, your room, and possibly the parking area, or reception area to reduce uncertainty and anxiety. The photos offer familiarity and take away any guessing or anticipation.

Autistic clients may stim (twirl hair, fiddle, bounce their legs up and down, rock, sway, or flap their hands, for example). This is for regulation and is calming. Try not to discourage stimming. You could instead provide items which provide sensory input to fiddle with, which might be soothing (not only for autistic people), or you could encourage them to bring their own.

Some autistic people can find it easier to draw, or create an image, or use photographs to communicate how they are feeling or what they are going through. However, some may also find this too abstract, but may find writing their thoughts down to be easier than speaking them.

The sensory environment in your room is important to consider. Avoid bright overhead lights and strong smells (room sprays or scented candles). Sensory overload can affect an autistic person's ability to concentrate, to communicate, and can increase their levels of distress. Similarly, face-to-face conversations can be too intense, so sitting sideways on, or engaging in a task together, may facilitate more relaxed communication. Also, check that the proximity you sit at is OK, as close proximity can cause distress or be overwhelming.

References

APA (2013). *Diagnostic and Statistical Manual of Mental Disorder*, Fifth Edition. Arlington, VA: American Psychiatric Association.

Anderson, D.K., Lord, C., Risi, S., DiLavore, P.S., Shulman, C., Thurm, A., Welch, K., and Pickles, A. (2007). Patterns of growth in verbal abilities among children with autism spectrum disorder. *Journal of Consulting and Clinical Psychology*, 75(4), p. 594–604. https://doi.org/10.1037/0022-006X.75.4.594

Au-Yeung, S.K., Bradley, L., Robertson, A.E., Shaw, R., Baron-Cohen, S., and Cassidy, S. (2019). Experience of mental health diagnosis and perceived misdiagnosis in autistic, possibly autistic and non-autistic adults. *Autism*, 23(6), p. 1508–1518. https://doi.org/10.1177/1362361318818167

Baldwin, S., and Costley, D. (2015). The experiences and needs of female adults with high-functioning autism spectrum disorder. *Autism*, 20(4), p. 483–495. https://doi.org/10.1177/1362361315590805

Balfe, M., and Tantam, D. (2010). A descriptive social and health profile of a community sample of adults and adolescents with Asperger syndrome. *BMC Research Notes*, 3, p. 300. http://www.biomedcentral.com/1756-0500/3/300

Behrman, R.E., and Butler, A.S. (Eds) (2007). *Preterm Birth: Causes, Consequences, and Prevention*. The National Academies Collection: Reports funded by National Institutes of Health. Washington, D.C.: National Academies Press.

Ben-Sasson, A., Hen, L., Fluss, R., Cermak, S.A., Engel-Yeger, B., and Gal, E. (2009). A meta-analysis of sensory modulation symptoms in individuals with autism spectrum disorders. *Journal of Autism and Developmental Disorders*. https://doi.org/10.1007/s10803-008-0593-3

Bird, G., and Cook, R. (2013). Mixed emotions: The contribution of alexithymia to the emotional symptoms of autism. *Translational Psychiatry*, *3*(7), p. e285–e285. https://doi.org/10.1038/tp.2013.61

Boland, H., DiSalvo, M., Fried, R., Woodworth, K.Y., Wilens, T., Faraone, S.V., and Biederman, J. (2020). A literature review and meta-analysis on the effects of ADHD medications on functional outcomes. *Journal of Psychiatric Research*, 123, p. 21–30. https://doi.org/10.1016/j.jpsychires.2020.01.006

Brinkman, S. (2016). *Diagnostic Cultures: A Cultural Approach to the Pathologization of Modern Life*. London, UK: Routledge.

Brugha, T.S., McManus, S., Bankart, J., Scott, F., Purdon, S., Smith, J., Bebbington, P., Jenkins, R., and Meltzer, H. (2011). The epidemiology of autism spectrum disorders in adults in the community in England. *Archives of General Psychiatry*, 68(5), p. 459–465. https://doi.org/10.10.1001/archgenpsychiatry.2011.38

Cambridge English Online Dictionary. (2021). Retrieved from https://dictionary.cambridge.org/dictionary/english/neurodivergent [accessed 12.12.21].

Cassidy, S., Bradley, P., Robinson, J., Allison, C., McHugh, M., and Baron-Cohen, S. (2014). Suicidal ideation and suicide plans or attempts in adults with Asperger's syndrome attending a specialist diagnostic clinic: A clinical cohort study. *The Lancet Psychiatry*, 1(2), p. 142–147. https://doi.org/10.1016/S2215-0366(14)70248-2

Courchesne, E., Campbell, K., and Solso, S. (2011). Brain growth across the life span in autism: Age specific changes in anatomical pathology. *Brain Research*, 1380, p. 138–145. https://doi.org/10.1016/j.brainres.2010.09.101

Devokut, J., Ende, D., Verhulst, C., Slappendel, G., Daalen, E., Maras, A., and Greaves-Lord, K. (2017). Factors influencing the probability of a diagnosis of autism spectrum disorder in girls versus boys. *Autism*, 21(6), p. 646–658. https://doi.org/10.1177/1362361316672178

Dudas, R.B., Lovejoy, C., Cassidy, S., Allison, C., Smith, P., and Baron-Cohen, S. (2017). The overlap between autistic spectrum conditions and borderline personality disorder. *PLoS ONE*, *12*(9), e0184447. https://doi.org/10.1371/journal.pone.0184447

Dugdale, A.-S., Thompson, A.R., Leedham, A., Beail, N., and Freeth, M. (2021). Intense connection and love: The experiences of autistic mothers. *Autism*, 25(7), p. 1973–1984. https://doi.org/10.1177/1362361321005987

Emerson, E. (2003). Mothers of children and adolescents with intellectual disability: Social and economic situation, mental health status, and the self–assessed social and psychological impact of the child's difficulties. *Journal of Intellectual Disability Research*, 47, p. 385–399. https://doi.org/10.1046/j.1365-2788.2003.00498.x

Haruvi-Lamden, N., Horesh, D., Zohar, S., Kraus, M., and Golan, O. (2020). Autism Spectrum Disorder and Post-Traumatic Stress Disorder: An unexplored co-occurrence of conditions. *Autism*, 24(4), p. 884–898. https://doi.org/10.1177/1362361320912143

Harwood, K., McLean, N., and Durkin, K. (2007). First-time mothers' expectations of parenthood: What happens when optimistic expectations are not matched by later experiences? *Developmental Psychology*, 43, p. 1–12. https://doi.org/10.1037/0012-1649.43.1.1

Hofvander, B., Delore, R., Chaste, P., Nydén, A., Wentz, E., Ståhlberg, O., Herbrecht, E., Stopin, A., Ankarsäter, H., Gillberg, C., Råstam, M., and Leboyer, M.

(2009). Psychiatric and psychosocial problems in adults with normal-intelligence autism spectrum disorders. *BMC Psychiatry*, 9, Article 35. https://doi.org/10.1186/1471-244X-9-35

Keuler, M.M., Schmidt, N.L., Van Hulle, C.A., Lemery-Chalfant, K., and Goldsmith, H.H. (2011). Sensory overresponsivity: Prenatal risk factors and temperamental contributions. *Journal of Developmental and Behavioral Paediatrics*, 32(7), p. 533–541. https://doi.org/10.1097/DBP.0b013e3182245c05

Kittel-Schneider, S., Quednow, B.B., Leutritz, A.L., McNeill, R.V., and Reif, A. (2021). Parental ADHD in pregnancy and the postpartum period – A systematic review. *Neuroscience and Biobehavioral Reviews*, 124, p. 63–77. https://doi.org/10.1016/j.neubiorev.2021.01.002

Kreiser, N.L., and White, S.W. (2014). ASD in females: Are we overstating the gender difference in diagnosis? *Clinical Child and Family Psychology Review*, 17, p. 67–84. https://doi.org/10.1007/s10567-013-0148-9

Lai, M.C., Kassee, C., Besney, R., Bonato, S., Hull, L., Mandy, W., Szatmari, P., and Ameis, S.H. (2019). Prevalence of co-occurring mental health diagnoses in the autism population: A systematic review and meta-analysis. *The Lancet Psychiatry*, 6(10), p. 819–829. https://doi.org/10.1016/S2215-0366(19)30289-5

LeFever Watson, G., Arcona, A.D., Antonuccio, D.O., and Healy, D. (2014). Shooting the messenger: The case of ADHD. *Journal of Contemporary Psychotherapy*, 44(1), p. 43–52. https://doi.org/10.1007/s10879-013-9244-x

Lin, L.Y. (2010). Factors associated with caregiving burden and maternal pessimism in mothers of adolescents with an autism spectrum disorder in Taiwan, *Occupational Therapy International*, 18, p. 96–105. https://doi.org/10.1002/oti.305

Lipinski, S., Boegl, K., Blanke, E.S., Suenkel, U., and Dziobek, I. (2021). A blind spot in mental healthcare? Psychotherapists lack education and expertise for the support of adults on the autism spectrum. *Autism*. https://doi.org/10.1177/13623613211057973

Milton, D. (2012). On the Ontological status of autism: The 'double empathy problem'. *Disability & Society*, 27(6), p. 883–887.

Nörby, U., Winbladh, B., and Källén, K. (2017). Perinatal outcomes after treatment with ADHD medication during pregnancy. *Pediatrics*, 140(6), p. e20170747. https://doi.org/10.1542/peds.2017-0747

Papadopoulos, D. (2021). Mothers' experiences and challenges raising a child with autism spectrum disorder: A qualitative study. *Brain Sciences*, 11(3), p. 309. https://doi.org/10.3390/brainsci11030309

Poulton, A.S., Armstrong, B., and Nanan, R.K. (2018). Perinatal outcomes of women diagnosed with attention-deficit/hyperactivity disorder: An Australian population-based cohort. *CNS Drugs*, 32, p. 377–386.

Raja, M. (2014). Suicide risk in adults with Asperger's syndrome. *The Lancet Psychiatry*, 1(2), p. 99–101. https://doi.org/10.1016/S2215-0366(14)70257-3

Reuben, K.E., Stanzione, C.M., and Singleton, J. (2021). Interpersonal trauma and posttraumatic stress in autistic adults. *Autism in Adulthood*, 3(3). https://doi.org/10.1089/aut.2020.0073

Roberts, A.L., Koenen, K.C., Lyall, K., Ascherio, A., and Weisskopf, M.G. (2014). Women's posttraumatic stress symptoms and autism spectrum disorder in their children. *Research in Autism Spectrum Disorders*, 8(6), p. 608–616. https://doi.org/10.1016/j.rasd.2014.02.004

Rumball, F., Happé, F., and Grey, N. (2020). Experience of trauma and PTSD symptoms in autistic adults: Risk of PTSD development following DSM-5 and non-DSM-5 traumatic life events. *Autism Research*, 12(12), p. 2122–2132. https://doi.org/10.1002/aur.2306

Singh, I. (2013). Brain talk: Power and negotiation in children's discourse about self, brain and behaviour. *Sociology of Health and Illness*, 35(6), p. 813–827. https://doi.org/10.1111/j.1467-9566.2012.01531

Sundeline, H., Stephansson, O., Hultman, M., and Ludvigsson, J. (2018). Pregnancy outcomes in women with autism: A nationwide population-based cohort study. *Clinical Epidemiology*, 10, p. 1817–1826. https://doi.org/10.2147/CLEP.S176910

Talcer, M.C., Duffy, O., and Pedlow, K. (2021). A qualitative exploration into the sensory experiences of autistic mothers. *Journal of Autism and Developmental Disorders*. https://doi.org/10.1007/s10803-021-05188-1

Top, D.N. Jr, Luke, S.G., Stephenson, K.G., and South, M. (2019). Psychophysiological arousal and auditory sensitivity in a cross-clinical sample of autistic and non-autistic anxious adults. *Frontiers in Psychiatry*, 9, p. 783. https://doi.org/10.3389/fpsyt.2018.00783

Uchida, N., Takahashi, K., Iwasaki, R., Yamada, R., Yoshimura, M., Endo, T.A., Kimura, S., Zhang, H., Nomoto, M., Tada, Y., Kinoshita, T., Itami, K., Hagihara, S., and Torii, K.U. (2018). Chemical hijacking of auxin signaling with an engineered auxin-TIR1 pair. *Nature Chemical Biology*, 14(3), p. 299–305.

Visser, S.N., Danielson, M.L., Bitsko, R.H., Holbrook, J.R., Kogan, M.D., Ghandour, R.M., Perou, R., and Blumberg, S.J. (2013). Trends in the parent-report of health care provider-diagnosed and medicated attention deficit/hyperactivity disorder: United States, 2003-2011. *Journal of the American Academy of Child and Adolescent Psychiatry*, 53(1), p. 34–46. https://doi.org/10.1016/j.jaac.2013.09.001

Wieland, N., Green, S., Ellingsen, R., and Baker, B.L. (2014). Parent–child problem solving in families of children with or without intellectual disability. *Journal of Intellectual Disability Research*, 58, p. 17–30. https://doi.org/10.1111/jir.12009

Zhu, Y., Liu, W., Li, Y., Wang, X., and Winterstein, A.G. (2017). Prevalence of ADHD in publicly insured adults. *Journal of Attention Disorders*. https://doi.org/10.1177/1087054717698815, 1087054717698815.

16 Couples Work

This is a short chapter on working with couples as I want to offer it as a plausible way of working. I do tend to see more women, men, husbands or partners on their own. However, I find working with the husband, partner and the couple really beneficial. Sometimes, the couple come because they are struggling with fertility issues or have experienced the loss of a baby. I also often ask the partner to come in for one or two sessions, so they can ask questions, allay fears and talk about some of the myths that may be prevalent to help in their knowledge and understanding of what is happening. Mostly, I find partners want to help in some way, or to know what they can do to have their partner back. It also gives me an opportunity to see how the couple interact. It is not at all unusual for me to receive an email or phone call from a concerned partner wanting to make an appointment for their partner to see me, sometimes without even consulting them. I am clear from the outset that the woman needs to contact me first. She needs to actually want to come to therapy; otherwise it is futile, particularly if she feels coerced into attending or if she is attending for the sake of her partner and not for herself.

I will split this chapter down into two sections. The first part looks at working with the partner for a session or two, normally in a psychoeducational way. The second part looks at working with couples who have approached me together. This is not about telling you how to work with couples; this is more about highlighting the positives that come from working with a couple, when they are facing some almost impossible challenges, such as those highlighted in Chapter 10.

Bringing the partner into the sessions

When a woman is unwell, her partner is often completely unsure of what is happening, and sometimes clueless that the woman is struggling with her mental health. Her behaviour can seem out of sorts, particularly if her anxiety is through the roof, and her partner may begin to question what on earth is going on. However, as I have said in various chapters of this book, some women are also so good at hiding their illness behind a mask of ok-ness. These women behave as if there is nothing wrong with them and are unable

DOI: 10.4324/9781003154891-18

to speak about their illness due to guilt and shame. In some instances, her partner may discount how she is feeling and will have expectations of her ability to cope that may be way in excess of what she can manage. It can come as a huge surprise to the partner that there is something wrong, although often they have a sense that something is going on.

If the partner is used to a woman who is normally independent and efficient, it can be particularly difficult for them to understand the fundamental changes that occur during pregnancy and childbirth. My role is to teach them that these changes are normal and natural. This can help partners come to terms with these changes and be more tolerant of them. Some partners don't quite seem to understand how the loss of autonomy a woman experiences and the total sense of responsibility for this tiny, screeching infant is all-consuming and terrifying. Being a partnership at this juncture in life together could have seemed to have a level of equality. However, no matter what, once a baby arrives, women seem to be expected to do the lion's share of the looking after. When the partner leaves for work, the ten to twelve hours of the day ahead can seem daunting and difficult. It can feel as though this is a period of servitude, where she needs to totally abnegate herself to the needs of the infant. Of course, this is totally true, and it does need to be this way, as the infant is totally vulnerable. This transition to becoming a mother is transformative, and not necessarily in a positive way. The term baby-centric sums it up: a time when everything else may seem to go out of the window.

Birth trauma is another area where the partner may value psychoeducation about what has happened, particularly if this plays a role in sexual dysfunction. It helps to engender empathy and for the other to become more realistic about their expectations of their partner and how to talk about this difficult subject without feeling pressured or ashamed. Elisabeth suffered quite severe physical birth trauma with her first child and unfortunately had to undergo several operations post-birth to rectify the damage. It affected her ability to care for her baby, as she found lifting, carrying and feeding her baby difficult. Physically, she was completely different to pre-birth. My role, as well as helping her to come to terms with the trauma, to help her with the flashbacks and debilitating night terrors, was also around helping her to unpick the shame and embarrassment she felt with her husband and the fact that she no longer wanted him to see her naked anymore. Laura felt disgusted with her body, the lack of control she had now had and her general feeling of discomfort which never went away. When we talked about sex, she was horrified at the thought of how this might happen, how she could even let her husband see the damage that giving birth had done to her. After a few weeks I asked her if her husband would attend some sessions with her so that he might begin to understand how she felt about her body and how it had let her down. Both in their early thirties, they had thought that sex was going to be an area that simply would no longer happen due to Laura's injuries. Gradually, over a period of some months, Laura began to come to terms with what had happened. Through reconstructive surgery, she was also able to finally begin to think about what it might be like to have intimacy with her husband again, and how they could both navigate their way through her trauma.

Mothers will often tell me things and then say: '*I have never told anyone this before*'. I wonder to myself why they have said nothing to their partner, their own mother, their friends, their health visitor. Bringing the partner in gives the mother an opportunity to voice how she is feeling, underneath the mask of being ok. This is not a therapy session for the partner. This is to help them understand what is going on, to put into context the woman's struggle, how she feels and how normal yet debilitating this may be. It is also an opportunity for the woman to ask for things from her partner, with a witness, that she may never have asked for before, such as help.

Some women are reticent about inviting their partners in. Will it change the dynamic between us (therapist and client)? Will it be useful? Will the partner feel 'got at' by me as the therapist? In response, I am curious if she wants to remain with her mask on, unable to admit to anyone but me just how bad she is feeling. Some women are also ashamed of their partner's lack of understanding and empathy. His reticence to come and have a session – why should he, there is nothing wrong with him - kind of attitude. Some women tell me their husbands simply won't understand that having a child is an everyday occurrence (female oriented, of course) and should not be blown out of proportion by a woman being overly dramatic. This only adds to my determination that the partner needs to come too, and quickly. These women know they are in a relationship of inequality from the outset.

My resolve is for partners to understand and acknowledge how unwell their wife/partner actually is, and to recognise that both their lives have now changed. Anna Machin has spent many years researching the role of fathers in the upbringing of their children and has written an excellent book called *The Life of Dad – the Making of the Modern Father*. This book lays out in detail the vital importance of a father's role and his fundamental contribution to the growth and development of his child. Machin's knowledge of genetics, neuroscience and psychology and can be really useful reading matter for a man who is ambivalent to his role of father. It is no longer an excuse that his wife is breastfeeding so he cannot help, or he does not know how to. This is a time for partnership, where both parties play a full role in the day-to-day care of their children. Yet still I see some men who are stuck in a time warp, where the expectation after the first two weeks of paternity leave is one of normal life: work, football, golf, the pub, a social life, home when he can – hopefully after the baby is in bed. This is a life where the expectation is that weekends will be for him to recover from work, with no real understanding that this is also what his partner wants too – a weekend to recover from single-parenting. A little psychoeducation can often go a long way to help with refocusing a man towards his wife and children.

Mostly, I find that partners who come to a session do want to know what they can do to help. Their lack of knowledge can be because their wife/partner has not actually been frank, open and honest about her illness.

Just one or two sessions are an invaluable time to help the couple bring their own psychological and emotional relief to each other. I always ensure the session is with both partners involved and I spend time before the joint session drawing out the minutiae of detail important to my client: how she expects the session to go; any fears she may have; what she wants me to say or highlight, so the session can be as effective as possible in bringing about the needed change.

Working with a couple

Couples work can be particularly helpful for those going through fertility difficulties, who have had a diagnosis of abnormalities in the fetus, or who are in the awful position of deciding whether to have a termination because of these abnormalities. Richard and Lucy were at different stages of grief and were experiencing heightened tension in their relationship. They had discovered their baby was not thriving in the womb due to an abnormality in its organs and had been informed that their baby might not survive birth. They were able to voice and explore their fears, expectations and grief, which were similar, but not the same. It was an opportunity to think about how they could tolerate the future together, as well as help them to grieve the loss of their 'perfect' baby. Another aspect of the work was helping them to form a united front to family and friends, who were not aware their baby's life was hanging by a thread. Richard knew his family did not deal with illness or disability well and he was struggling with the lack of compassion he was sure they would receive once his family heard. We spent time exploring how Richard and Lucy could field difficult questions and how Richard might step into the silent void of his family's lack of emotional awareness. Lucy struggled with responding from a non-defensive position. She was angry that Richard's family were incapable of offering support and empathy when the couple were going through such a tough time. Helping them both with strategies of response helped them both to feel more in control of their intense distress and grief.

Couples work is no different in parenthood. Most often it is the lack of connection or the break in connection that is placing strain on the relationship. Finding the commonality is often really important, rather than focusing on the negative aspects. I have found it useful to have a supervisor who is familiar with this type of work and who helps to bring out any unconscious bias towards one or other of the party.

Working with a couple to help with parent/infant bonding is an enjoyable aspect of the work. This can be partly psychoeducational, helping the couple to understand why parent–infant bonding is so crucial to the infant's well-being. It can also be about helping the couple to decipher what may be going on with their infant and how to recognise particular cues such as certain types of crying and behaviour. I worked with Tom and May after the birth of their twins and May's subsequent psychosis and stay in an inpatient mother and baby unit. May had rejected her babies, but in particular, she rejected her daughter. When I asked May about her daughter Bethan, May told me that Bethan would turn her head away from her whenever May looked at her. I asked her to show me what was happening with Bethan and sure enough, when May popped her on the floor and began to interact with her, Bethan turned her face to the side. 'See, I told you, she does not like me' May said in distress. I was able to talk May through how some babies can feel overwhelmed with eye-to-eye contact and will turn their head away as a way to break the intensity. I explained to her that this was not a sign of rejection, more a sign that Bethan was finding May's intensity a little too much. Tom was able to let me know that he had noticed May being so determined to 'win' Bethan over that May was, on occasion, seeming a little too fixated on Bethan. We talked together about May's experience. How upset she felt at this rejection. It led to a really fruitful session unpicking May's intense relationship with her own mother, which, in May's words, was dysfunctional. May began to understand that the rejection she felt from Bethan was similar to the rejection May experienced from her mother. She also began to realise that Bethan was not rejecting her. Instead May talked about how uncomfortable she felt when her mother gave her 'one of her looks', an intensity that May said was almost unbearable when she was a child. We explored how May might be less intense with her daughter, that she could choose to be different to her mother and not offer Bethan the 'same' experience, but something different and more appropriate.

Conclusion

Couples work can be really beneficial as it can help the couple to reconnect rather than split apart due to the challenges they are facing. It is no different from any other type of couples work and training in the transferential dynamics as well as understanding how the couple function together due to their attachment styles is both useful and necessary as the work always stimulates transference.

17 Conventional Treatment of Maternal Mental Illness

This chapter looks briefly at the conventional type of psychotropic drug usage for maternal mental illness. The purpose is to give information about the type of medication and the statistics on usage, as well as some of the research on abnormalities that may occur with some forms of medication. There will be many times when women I am treating are taking psychotropic medication in addition to their therapy. I have found it useful to know about some of the research that exists so that I am more informed about the type of medication, the side effects on mother and fetus/infant and how I might support those women who no longer wish to take their medication, as they are finding the benefits are heavily outweighed by the more negative effects the drugs have. For a more in-depth look at psychiatric drugs please see Joanna Moncrieff's book *Psychiatric Drugs: The Truth about How They Work and How to Come Off Them*. Although Moncrieff is not specifically looking at drug usage in pregnancy and postnatally, her writing is nonetheless informative and helpful.

Generally, there has been a doubling of medication usage in the last 20 years. At present, around one in ten young women are prescribed antidepressants in healthcare settings (Boyd, et al., 2015; Kantor et al., 2015). This is troubling as it would appear that psychotropic medication is being overused in women who might benefit from psychological therapy as a suitable alternative. There may also be underuse (Yonkers et al., 2011) or even a discontinuation in those women who have a diagnosis such as bipolar disorder (Cohen et al., 2006; Wesseloo et al., 2016).

Antidepressants continue to be the first type of treatment in the perinatal period (Meunier, Bennett & Coco, 2013; Yonkers et al., 2009). Around 2–3% of women take antidepressants in pregnancy and this increases to between 5% and 7% after birth. Yet, there is evidence that these drugs pass through both the placenta and breast milk (Dubovicky et al., 2017). There is also disagreement about the effects of psychotropic drugs used both in the antenatal and postnatal period. Controversy arises because of possible side effects on both mother and baby (Galbally et al., 2009; Lugo-Candelas et al., 2018; Rosenquist, 2013). For breastfeeding mothers, a decision on whether to take medication is influenced by the woman's knowledge of and concerns about

DOI: 10.4324/9781003154891-19

infant exposure to medication via breast milk (Chabrol et al., 2004; Epperson et al., 2003; Kim, O'Reardon & Epperson, 2010; Pearlstein et al., 2006).

Selective serotonin reuptake inhibitors (SSRIs) have recently caused controversy. Recently an infant's exposure to SSRIs as a fetus, and its brain structure and connectivity once born, was shown to have a negative correlation, and the conclusion drawn was that the SSRI exposure in pregnancy was associated with brain development, particularly in emotional processing, causing an increase in susceptibility to anxiety and depression in the infant (Lugo-Candelas et al., 2018).

Zoloft (known as Sertraline in the UK) was the subject of a lawsuit regarding birth defects after its usage in pregnancy (Mehrotra, 2016). Fluoxetine is also subject to concerns following reports of increased risk of cardiac malformations in the infant if used during pregnancy, although one study concludes that there is no increased risk (Riggin et al., 2013). Fluoxetine is also associated with increased risk of the fetus developing Autism Spectrum Disorder (Gentile, 2015; Man et al., 2015), or atrial/ventricular defects and craniosynostosis (Bérard, Zhao & Sheehy, 2015). Pregabalin usage in the first trimester of pregnancy has been shown to result in the risk of increased major birth defects (Winterfeld et al., 2016). Rosenquist (2013) has raised concerns about the dependency arising from the usage of SSRIs, the difficulty of withdrawal and the increased knowledge of toxicity. There is also concern about the effects of 'neonatal serotonin discontinuation syndrome' (Galbally et al., 2009). Women can find themselves in a difficult bind of choosing between accepting pharmacotherapy treatment that may be harmful to themselves or their child, or possibly no treatment at all (Freeman, 2009; Wisner et al., 2000).

Use of antipsychotics in pregnancy doubled in the decade to 2016 (Huybrechts et al., 2016). There would appear to be little data on antipsychotics and their efficacy or safety in the postnatal period. Taylor, Stewart and Howard in a study using electronic medical records did not appear to find evidence that antipsychotics were a protective factor for women with psychosis in the first three months after birth (2019). Huybrechts et al. found that antipsychotic use did not meaningfully increase the risk of cardiac or congenital malformations, although Risperidone needs more research as it did show a small increase (2016).

In a small study of women offered psychotherapy and/or Sertraline, women who were breastfeeding were less likely to choose Sertraline over psychotherapy (Pearlstein et al., 2006). In the UK, funding for treatment other than psychotropic medication is limited by the National Health Service, although there is now a strategy to tackle gaps in service provision (NHS England, 2018). Treatment strategies recommended in NICE guidelines (2015) were either pharmacotherapy, or Cognitive Behavioural Treatment (CBT), offered often through the IAPT service. However, in the most recent guidelines it would appear that only pharmacotherapy is now recommended (NICE, 2020). Worldwide, Davies, Rahman and Lund (2019) suggest the scaling up of evidence-based psychotherapy for perinatal mental disorders in low-and middle-income countries. Although the authors say such services do need to be tailored to the local contexts. Research shows that the perceived relevance of treatment is critical to engagement and treatment adherence, as is perinatal specific content, which may influence the attrition rates for treatment, which are high (O'Mahen et al., 2015).

A large-scale qualitative study of the experience and attributions of post-natal depression found that 'talking therapies' were the preference of women, in a cross-cultural study incorporating 11 countries (Austria, France, Ireland, Italy, Japan, Portugal, Sweden, Switzerland, United States, Uganda and UK) (Oates et al., 2004). This study found participants did not universally recognise a need for medical intervention, viewing the causes and remedies as lying in the psychosocial domain. Goodman (2009) also found a high level (92%) of preference for psychotherapy as a treatment option for depression in pregnancy, which concurs with studies into patient preferences in primary care for depression (Backenstrass et al., 2006; Dwight-Johnson et al., 2000; van Shaik et al., 2004).

Conclusion

It would appear that psychotherapy is a more preferable option to psycho-tropic medication for women in pregnancy and childbirth. However, this form of treatment is not commonly available yet, as a first line of treatment. This makes it difficult for women to make an informed choice for treatment, as they may well be choosing between only medication or no treatment at all. Increase in choice is vital for women and where possible, it would appear sensible to avoid all medication in pregnancy due to the incomplete knowledge of their safety and the risk posed towards the fetus.

References

Backenstrass, M., Joest, K., Frank, A., Hingmann, S., Mundt, C., and Kronmüller, K.T. (2006). Preferences for treatment in primary care: A comparison of nondepressive, sub-syndromal and major depressive patients. *General Hospital Psychiatry*, 28(2), p. 178–180. https://doi.org/10.1016/j.genhosppsych.2005.10.001

Bérard, A., Zhao, J.-P., and Sheehy, O. (2015). Sertraline use during pregnancy and the risk of major malformations. *American Journal of Obstetrics and Gynecology*, 212(6), p. 795.E1–795.E12. https://doi.org/10.1016/j.ajog.2015.01.034

Boyd, A., Van de Velde, S., Pivette, M., Ten Have, M., Florescu, S., O'Neill, S., Caldas-de-Almeida, J.M., Vilagut, G., Haro, J.M., Alonso, J., and Kovess-Masféty, V.; EU-WMH investigators. (2015). Gender differences in psychotropic use across Europe: Results from a large cross-sectional, population-based study. *European Psychiatry*, 30(6), p. 778–788. https://doi.org/10.1016/j.eurpsy.2015.05.001, Epub 2015 Jun 4. PMID: 26052073.

Chabrol, H., Teissedre, F., Armitage, J., Danel, M., and Walburg, V. (2004). Acceptability of psychotherapy and antidepressants for postnatal depression among newly delivered mothers. *Journal of Reproductive and Infant Psychology*, 22, p. 5–12. https://doi.org/10.10 80/02646830310001643094

Cohen, L.S., Altshuler, L.L., and Harlow, B.L., et al. (2006). Relapse of major depression during pregnancy in women who maintain or discontinue antidepressant treatment *JAMA*, 295(5), p. 499–507. https://doi.org/10.1001/jama.295.5.499

Davies, T., Rahman, A., and Lund, C. (2019). Psychotherapy for perinatal mental disorders in low- and middle-income countries. In Dan J. Stein, Judith K. Bass & Stefan G. Hofmann (Eds.), *Global Mental Health in Practice, Global Mental Health and Psychotherapy*, p. 301–319. Academic Press. https://doi.org/10.1016/B978-0-12-814932-4.00014-8

Dubovicky, M., Belovicova, K., Csatlosova, K., and Bogi, E. (2017). Risks of using SSRI/SNRI antidepressants during pregnancy and lactation. *Interdisciplinary Toxicology*, 10(1), p. 30–34. https://doi.org/10.1515/intox-2017-0004

Dwight-Johnson, M., Sherbourne, C.D., Liao, D., and Wells, K.B. (2000). Treatment preferences among depressed primary care patients. *Journal of General Internal Medicine*, 15(8), p. 527–534. https://doi.org/10.1046/j.1525-1497.2000.08035.x

Epperson, C.N., Jatlow, P.I., Czarkowski, K., and Anderson, G.M. (2003). Maternal fluoxetine treatment in the postpartum period: Effects on platelet serotonin and plasma drug levels in breastfeeding mother-infant pairs. *Pediatrics*, 112, p. e425–e429. https://doi.org/10.1542/peds.112.5.e425

Freeman, M.P. (2009). Perinatal psychiatry: The challenges of making rational treatment decisions at the interface of psychiatry and obstetrics. *Journal of Clinical Psychiatry*, 70(9), p. 1311–1312. https://doi.org/10.4088/JCP.09f05512

Galbally, M., Lewis, A.J., Lum, J., and Buist, A. (2009). Serotonin discontinuation syndrome following in utero exposure to antidepressant medication: A prospective study. *Australian and New Zealand Journal of Psychiatry*, 43, p. 846–854. https://doi.org/10.1080/00048670903107583

Gentile, S. (2015). Prenatal antidepressant exposure and the risk of autism spectrum disorders in children. Are we looking at the fall of Gods? *Journal of Affective Disorders*, 182, p. 132–137. https://doi.org/10.1016/j.jad.2015.04.048

Goodman, J.H. (2009). Women's attitudes, preferences, and perceived barriers to treatment for perinatal depression. *Birth*, 36(1), p. 60–69. https://doi.org/10.1111/j.1523-536X.2008.00296.x

Huybrechts, K.F., Hernández-Díaz, S., Patorno, E., Desai, R.J., Mogun, H., Dejene, S.Z., Cohen, J.M., Panchaud, A., Cohen, L., and Bateman, B.T. (2016). Antipsychotic use in pregnancy and the risk for congenital malformations. *JAMA Psychiatry*, 73(9), p. 938–946. https://doi.org/10.1001/jamapsychiatry.2016.1520

Kantor, E.D., Rehm, C.D., Haas, J.S., Chan, A.T., and Giovannucci, E.L. (2015). Trends in prescription drug use among adults in the United States from 1999–2012. *JAMA*, 314(17), p. 1818–1831. https://doi.org/10.1001/jama.2015.13766

Kim, D.R., O'Reardon, J.P., and Epperson, C.N. (2010). Guidelines for the management of depression during pregnancy. *Current Psychiatry Reports*, 12, p. 279–281. https://doi.org.10.1007/s11920-010-0114-x

Lugo-Candelas, C., Cha, J., and Hong, S., et al. (2018). Associations between brain structure and connectivity in infants and exposure to selective serotonin reuptake inhibitors during pregnancy. *JAMA Pediatrics*, published online 9 April 2018. https://doi.org/10.1001/jamapediatrics.2017.5227

Man, K.K.C., Tong, H.H.Y., Wong, L.Y.L., Chan, E.W., Simonoff, E., and Wong, I.C.K. (2015). Exposure to selective serotonin reuptake inhibitors during pregnancy and risk of autism spectrum disorder in children: A systematic review and meta-analysis of observational studies. *Neuroscience & Biobehavioral Reviews*, 49, p. 82–89. https://doi.org/10.1016/j.neubiorev.2014.11.020

Mehrotra, K. (2016) Pfizer wins dismissal in Zoloft birth defect warning cases. Bloomberg Businessweek, https://www.bloomberg.com/news/article/2016-04-06/Pfizer-wins-dismissal-in-zoloft-birth-defect-warning-cases

Meunier, M.R., Bennett, I.M., and Coco, A.S. (2013). Use of antidepressant medication in the United States during pregnancy, 2002-2010. *Psychiatric Services – Brief Reports, pl.psychiatryonline.org*, 64(11), p. 1157–1160. https://www.researchgate.net/profile/Ian-Bennett-5/publication/258253260_Use_of_Antidepressant_Medication_in_the_United_States_During_Pregnancy_2002-2010/links/567d927608aebccc4e040389/Use-of-Antidepressant-Medication-in-the-United-States-During-Pregnancy-2002-2010.pdf

National Institute for Health and Care Excellence. (2015). *Antenatal and Postnatal Mental Health: Clinical Management and Service Guidance.* Retrieved from https://www.guidelines.co.uk/NICE/Postnatal-mental-health/252557.article [accessed 18.12.21].

National Institute for Health and Care Excellence (2020). *Antenatal and Postnatal Mental Health: Clinical Management and Service Guidance.* Retrieved from https://www.guidelines.co.uk/mental-health/nice-antenatal-and-postnatal-mental-health-guideline/252557.article [accessed 18.12.21].

NHS England. (2018). *The Perinatal Mental Health Care Pathways.* Retrieved from https://www.england.nhs.uk/wp-content/uploads/2018/05/perinatal-mental-health-care-pathway.pdf [accessed 18.12.21].

Oates, M.R., Cox, J.L., Neema, S., Asten, P., Glangeaud-Freudenthal, N., Figueiredo, B., Gorman, L.L., Hacking, S., Hirst, E., Martin, H., Kammerer, C., Klier, M., Seneviratne, G., Smith, M., Sutter-Dally, A.-L., Valoriani, V., Wickberg, B., and Yoshida, K. (2004). Postnatal depression across countries and cultures: A qualitative study. *British Journal of Psychiatry*, 184(46), p. s10–s16 https://doi.org/10.1192/bjp.184.46.s10

O'Mahen, H.A., Grieve, H., Jones, J., McGinley, J., Woodford, J., and Wilkinson, E. (2015). Women's experiences of factors affecting treatment engagement and adherence in internet delivered behavioural activation for postnatal depression. *Internet Interventions*, 2(1), p. 84–90. https://doi.org/10.1016/j.invent.2014.11.003

Pearlstein, T.N., Zlotnick, C., Battle, C.L., Stuart, S., O'Hara, M.W., Price, A.B., Grause, M.A., and Howard, M. (2006). Patient choice of treatment for postpartum depression: A pilot study. *Archive of Women's Mental Health,* 9, p. 303–308. https://doi.org/10.1007/s00737-006-0145-9

Riggin, L., Frankel, Z., Moretti, M., Pupco, A., and Koren, G. (2013). MOTHERISK ROUNDS: The fetal safety of fluoxetine: A systematic review and meta-analysis. *Journal of Obstetrics and Gynaecology Canada*, 35(4), p. 362–369. https://doi.org/10.1016/S1701-2163(15)30965-8

Rosenquist, S.E. (2013). When the bough breaks: Rethinking treatment strategies for perinatal depression. *American Journal of Clinical Hypnosis*, 55, p. 291–323. https://doi.org/10.1080/00029157.2012.723284

Taylor, C.L., Stewart, R.J., and Howard, L.M. (2019). Relapse in the first three months postpartum in women with history of serious mental illness. *Schizophrenia Research*, 204, p. 46–54. https://doi.org/10.1016/j.schres.2018.07.037, Epub 2018 Aug 5. PMID: 30089534.

van Shaik, D.J., Klijn, A.F., van Hout, H.P., van Marwijk, H.W., Beekman, A.T., de Haan, M., and van Dyck, R. (2004). Patients' preferences in the treatment of depressive disorder in primary care. *General hospital Psychiatry*, 26, p. 184–189. https://doi.org/10.1016/j.genhosppsych.2003.12.001

Wesseloo, R., Kamperman, A.M., Munk-Olsen, T., Pop, V.J., Kushner, S.A., and Bergink, V. (2016). Risk of postpartum relapse in bipolar disorder and postpartum psychosis: A systematic review and meta-analysis. *American Journal of Psychiatry*, 173, 117–127. https://doi.org/10.1176/appi.ajp.2015.15010124

Winterfeld, U., Merlob, P., Baud, D., Rousson, V., Panchaud, A., Rothuizen, L.E., Bernard, N., Vial, T., Yates, L.M., Pistelli, A., Ellfolk, M., Eleftheriou, G., de Vries, L.C., Jonville-Bera, A.-P., Kadioglu, J., Biollaz, J., and Buclin, T. (2016). Pregnancy outcome following maternal exposure to pregabalin may call for concern. *Neurology*. https://doi.org/10.1212/WNL.0000000000002767

Wisner, K.L., Zarin, D.A., Holmboe, E.S., Appelbaum, P.S., Gelenberg, A.J., Leonard, H.L., and Frank, E. (2000). Risk-benefit decision making for treatment of depression during pregnancy. *American Journal of Psychiatry*, 157, p. 1933–1940. https://doi.org/10.1176/appi.ajp.157.12.1933

Yonkers, K.A., Wisner, K.L., Stewart, D.E., Oberlander, T.F., Dell, D.L., Stotland, N., Ramin, S., Chaudron, L., and Lockwood, C. (2009). The management of depression during pregnancy: A report from the American Psychiatric Association and the American College of Obstetricians and Gynecologists. *Obstetrics and Gynecology*, 114(3), p. 703–713.

Yonkers, K.A., Gotman, N., Smith, M.V., Forray, A., Belanger, K., Brunetto, W.L., Lin, H., Burkman, R.T., Zelop, C.M., and Lockwood, C.J. (2011). Does antidepressant use attenuate the risk of a major depressive episode in pregnancy? *Epidemiology*, 22(6), p. 848–854. https://doi.org/10.1097/EDE.0b013e3182306847, PMID: 21900825; PMCID: PMC3188383.

18 A Lifetime Reduction in Mental Illness?

Maternal mental illness not only affects the woman, her fetus/infant and her family, it touches all of us, as it is so far reaching. So many women experience some form of mental illness at this time and statistics are not and never will be representative as many women never speak of it, and never ask for help. Maternal mental illness is also transgenerational in its nature. Often, the woman's mother and grandmother will have experienced something similar and have their own traumatic birth stories.

We already know the impact and damage stress has on the body and the mind-body link between mental health disorders and our physical ailments such as cancer, diabetes, heart disease (Maté, 2019; Stein et al., 2019). Why would it be any different for a woman and her fetus/infant if she is experiencing stress or distress? If maternal mental illness stems from a woman's past history, particularly from relational trauma or historical mental illness, it is possible that treating women at this time could offer longer term benefits such as mental and physical health. Certainly, in the work I have done, clients have told me they no longer feel the way they did prior to psychotherapy. Something has altered beneficially, which has had a long-lasting impact on the woman, her child and her family.

Some of the long-term benefits of addressing the cause of maternal mental illness are:

- Changes in attachment style
- Relational connection
- Reduction in trauma, shame and stigma
- Attunement
- Self-care
- Becoming the 'good enough' mother

Each one of these aspects is part of maternal wellness and comes together to form the resilience a woman needs to raise her children and lead a life without trauma, shame, stigma and silence, a life she can enjoy.

These six aspects do not preclude the possibility that hormones also play a role in maternal mental illness. This makes sense, although we do not

DOI: 10.4324/9781003154891-20

yet know the role they play through pregnancy and post birth. It is possible that hormones cause an exacerbation of underlying mental conditions, which when combined with the normal stresses of childbirth and lack of sleep form this perfect storm of distress. We do know that the brain goes through particular changes on a physiological and behavioural level and that brain plasticity changes during pregnancy and lactation (Hillerer et al., 2014). However, little research has been conducted on hormonal changes within pregnancy and post birth. What research has been done has advocated pharmacological substances as treatment (Trifu, Vladuti & Popescu, 2019).

Changes in attachment style

If a woman comes with an insecure attachment style there is always the potential for her to experience something different, to receive a new style of relating, one in which the therapist is able to tolerate, be affected by and impacted by her. Attachment provides the safety and security that she may never have experienced before. Humans are hard-wired to seek comfort and security and attachment is our way of ensuring our comfort and security; it is a biological process. Human survival is predicated on attachment and relationship. In relational psychotherapy we are working with the potentiality of relationship, attachment and proximity/closeness, as this is the part that is fundamental for change in the client.

This attachment relationship is one in which the relational therapist is promoting mentalizing or reflective functioning (being able to understand one's own, and others', internal space of emotions, motivating factors, thoughts, transferences). This is not only useful for helping women to regulate their emotions but affords awareness of emotions whilst still remaining in the emotion (Bateman & Fonagy, 2006). For a modern theory of attachment in its entirety, please see Schore (2017).

Relational connection

Relational connection is the most important aspect of healing in psychotherapy because the fundamental experience of deep relational connectedness offers a bidirectional transformative experience, for client and therapist. Deep relational connection is about being vulnerable to everything the relationship will bring – feelings, not knowing, not understanding, as well as anxieties, discomfort, spontaneity and authenticity – remaining in the relationship, no matter how difficult it can become, metabolising the feelings, experiencing the processes and enactments, transforming the implicit presymbolic experiences into ones that can be spoken and integrated. This type of psychotherapy is about being open to the reality of relationship, to know and understand that it will never be perfect, mistakes will be made, yet knowing, trusting and experiencing the transformative effect of a healthy, new response from an engaged and interested other. Research is also showing us that it is the unconscious elements (on an implicit/automatic level) that are much more important than the conscious aspects of dysregulation of emotion (Gyurak, Gross & Etkin, 2011).

In relational psychotherapy we are working similarly to the role of the mother with her newborn or young infant. She is metabolising the infant's difficult and unpleasant emotions and feelings. We may also need to be metabolising the adult's difficult and unpleasant emotions and feelings, because the original mother/caregiver was unable to offer this and because the client has found that her mental illness has been re-evoked in the process of becoming a mother. Working with maternal mental illness is close to working with the traces of the borderspace (Ettinger, 2006), with subjectivity as encounter – intrapsychic, intersubjective and transubjective. It is in this space where the 'unthought known' (Bollas, 1987, p 4) becomes the thought known in the space of event-encounter (Ettinger, 2006). Ettinger believes that if these traces of the borderspace go unrecognised: *'the traces will haunt the subject in a variety of symbolically foreclosed but affectively pressing ways, such as hallucinations, displaced phantasies, or uncanny moments'* (p. 16.7). I believe these traces of the borderspace can be re-evoked in maternal mental illness.

As a relational psychotherapist working with maternal mental illness, I am always asking myself am I accessible to my client, am I responsive to her, am I fully engaged with her story, am I able to meet her right brain to right brain, in a way that helps her experience dysregulation in a tolerable way with me as co-regulator.

Above all, nearly every mother wants to feel ok so that she can concentrate on building and developing the relationship she has with her infant and her family. We all need good connections for wellbeing, both intrapsychically, within ourselves, and also interpersonally, with others.

Reduction in trauma, shame and stigma

Maternal mental illness is not a disease, nor is it a chemical imbalance in our brains. It stems from a multitude of factors, one of which is relational trauma. This type of trauma is unique to each and every single mother. Every woman I see has a relational lack, or missing element. And from childhood her life has become about seeking out the lack – unconsciously searching for and finding those who might fit a representation of her lack. Thus, begins the repeating relational patterns. Humans are often unaware of why they keep repeating these patterns and the deep compulsion we all have to repair our earliest fractured relationships. Relational psychotherapy can help the woman to understand what she is seeking out or searching for, and what she is actually needing, which for many is the need for connection, safety and security,

The feelings of stigma and shame are culturally and societally constructed and are engendered in women due to their sense of not fitting the stereotype of the 'mother' figure that is mythologised within society, culture and religion. The woman may find it difficult to adapt to this 'lack' in herself and may find she is pulled in many ways, such as trying to be the perfect mother and yet also needing to provide financially for her family.

Trauma, shame and stigma are parts of this illness that are fixable. Interventions are possible within health care systems, and input from mothers themselves would improve shame and stigma-related knowledge and attitudes. Early intervention, at those critical stages of an infant's brain growth, can change the transgenerational transmission of relational trauma and mental illness. Cultural and societal knowledge of this transmission can offer future parent's choices in their decision-making processes. At present, women do not seem able to speak of their experiences of shame and stigma, and their voices have, as yet, not been clearly heard.

Attunement

The therapeutic role includes being attuned to our client implicitly, but why is attunement so important in psychotherapy? For much the same reason as it is so important to an infant. If the other is not attuned to us, then we find it difficult to know who we are or how we are doing. We rely on the other to mirror this to us. Without it, there is nothingness; we know nothing about who we are. For those adults who have struggled in life without the attunement from their caregiver, there is often this sense of a black hole of nothingness. When we attempt to fill that black hole ourselves, we tend to place negativity into it.

When there is stuckness, or ambivalence in the therapeutic relationship, attunement helps us to recognise and attend to it. Our client's experience is unique and when she is stuck this may be a reflection on her and on the therapy, and a lack in the therapeutic alliance. Staying attuned can help us gain a sense of when we are heading towards a dead end.

Self-care

Many women find self-care such a difficult concept, possibly because they are hard-wired to always be thinking about the other.

WHO define self-care as: '*The ability of individuals, families and communities to promote health, prevent disease, maintain health, and to cope with illness and disability with or without the support of a healthcare provider*' (2021). Self-care is not selfishness, nor is it self-serving. It is the ability to place our own mental and physical wellbeing at the forefront of our agenda. It is us who determine our own behaviour regarding self-care. Mothers need to prioritise themselves, in order to be able to look after the wellbeing of their children and family, to act, rather than react to healthcare needs. Using the metaphor of the oxygen mask in an airplane: mothers need to attend to their own self-care needs first to be able to adequately help their children. A mother who is unable to prioritise her own needs will struggle with the needs of others and quickly become exhausted and overwhelmed.

The 'Good enough' mother

In contrast to the 'perfect' mother, who cannot exist because no mother can attend to their baby's needs all of the time, the good enough mother is one who can be sensitive, empathic and compassionate to her child, is emotionally and physically responsive and available, provides a safe, secure environment and is attuned and adapted to the experiences of her baby. However, she does not try to stop her baby from experiencing difficult emotions as she knows that it is important for her baby to experience negative feelings and to learn how to tolerate frustration. Winnicott (1953) was the first to delineate what a 'good enough' mother is and used this title, the good enough mother, to explain how babies and children need their mothers to fail them regularly in ways that the child finds tolerable. When this happens, a child will experience frustration and will be able to gradually accept disillusionment. As the child grows up the child will be able to transition to a more autonomous position, a person who is not dependent always on the 'other'. The Center on the Developing Child at Harvard University has researched what they call 'serve and return' as a capacity building environment and shows how essential this is for the child's growing brain capacity for toleration.

Unfortunately, many women hear the term 'good enough mother' and interpret this to mean that this is not enough, that the only way is to be a perfect mother, putting so much pressure on themselves to be more than for their child. However, this ends up backfiring, as the child ends up delicate and fragile and unable to tolerate any kind of disappointment in life, or alternatively, who believes that the whole world revolves around them. Other mothers may hear that they do not need to attend to their children, and that the television or video games are enough. However, this can leave the child with a lack of human connection. There is a fine balance between the two extremes.

Final thoughts

It is our diversity that is the wonder of human beings. When we give birth, we give life and there is untold possibility and potential in that new, naked, screeching infant. Yet, from the moment a woman conceives she risks negative exposure, particularly from the pain of judgement. There is possibly no other part of life in which women lay themselves quite so bare to criticism from the 'other'. And if there is no criticism, women will engender it internally to punish themselves.

Mellacqua, in his book on the Transactional Analysis of Schizophrenia says of mental health that it is '*fundamentally family, social, organizational, and even "political" health (from the Greek polis for "city" or "community"), with profound implications for an entire community (large or small) of individuals*' (2021, p. 23). Maternal mental illness is a societal problem and the focus of our lens needs to be directed towards the future generations. As Weinstein says: '*The opportunity to optimally support the health and well-being of women, girls, any partners they may have and their offspring in current and future generations hinges on the global acknowledgement of the critical impacts of our experiences during the prenatal period*' (2016, p. 270). As yet, governments and society do not take this illness seriously enough.

In many of the chapters in this book I have only been able to touch on some aspects of maternal mental illness and motherhood, such as working with creativity and creative techniques, neurodivergence and narratives of maternal mental illness. Fathers and partners are also far too absent in the book, as are same-sex couples and adoptive parents. There are so many other aspects that compound this illness or parts of family systems that are impacted by it, which I have not had space to mention, such as the impact on the siblings, and the impact on the infant of surrogacy and adoption. Then there is displacement due to economic reasons; or the trauma of war and the impact on pregnant women and children. What about raising children in a culture which is not your own; the impact on the family, women and children when there is regime change, and the families are split apart such as in Afghanistan in August of 2021. What about COVID-19 and the pandemic, and its impact on pregnancy, birth and families. There are so much more to say and so many more aspects that need to be researched.

The main aim of this book has been to highlight the depth and breadth of maternal mental illness, to impart knowledge about women's experiences of it, what women are likely to bring to psychotherapy, and how we can treat them. It is also to highlight that the term postnatal depression falls so short of describing what this actually is. I want everyone to understand that this is a personal form of illness, and that mothers do not fit some specific formula. Nor is there a magic pill that can take it away. I want everyone to realise how detrimental the impact of this illness can be, that it is transgenerational and can cause lifelong mental illness for the infant too. Yet it does not need to be detrimental; it is treatable.

My aim has also been to highlight how relational psychotherapy can be a useful and beneficial form of treatment, impacting the mother, the infant, the family and also the economy. Relational psychotherapy is a process of weaving a web of relational meaning, often where there was no such meaning before, to allow the mother to explore, discover and become really aware of who she is, how she is and how she operates in the world with others. It is also a process of interweaving this new meaning into her old one.

Every fetus leaves microchimeric fetal cells as a trace of connection within their mother, some lasting for decades (Dawe, Tan & Xiao, 2007). Vice versa, every fetus, from conception onwards, is connected to the 'Other' and cannot be in life without the Other, and still holds traces of them in their body. Relational trauma also leaves traces, scars and shadows which continue to persist. I hope that after relational psychotherapy, something exists of the good-enough therapist within the client, a trace the woman can take with her into her future healthier life.

References

Bateman, A.W., and Fonagy, P. (2006). *Mentalization-Based Treatment for Borderline Personality Disorder: A Practical Guide.* Oxford, UK: Oxford University Press.

Bollas, C. (1987). *The Shadow of The Object – Psychoanalysis of the Unthought Known.* New York: Columbia University Press.

Dawe, G.S., Tan, X.W., and Xiao, Z.-C. (2007). Cell migration from baby to mother. *Cell Adhesion & Migration*, 1(1), p. 19–27. Epub 2007 Jan 28. PMID: 19262088; PMCID: PMC2633676.

Ettinger, B.L. (2006). *The Matrixial Borderspace.* Minneapolis, MN: The University of Minnesota Press.

Gyurak, A., Gross, J.J., and Etkin, A. (2011). Explicit ad implicit emotion regulation: A dual-process framework. *Cognition & Emotion*, 25, p. 400–412. https://doi.org/10. 1080/02699931.2010.544160

Hillerer, K.M., Jacobs, V.R., Fischer, T., and Aigner, L. (2014). The maternal brain: An organ with peripartal plasticity. *Neural Plasticity*, 574159. https://doi.org/10.1155/ 2014/574159

Maté, G. (2019). *When the Body Says No: The Cost of Hidden Stress.* London: Vermillion.

Mellacqua, Z. (2021). *Transactional Analysis of Schizophrenia: The Naked Self.* Abingdon, UK: Routledge.

Schore, A.N. (2017). Modern attachment theory. In S.N. Gold (Ed), *APA Handbook of Trauma Psychology: Foundations in Knowledge.* pp. 339–406. Washington, DC: American Psychological Association.

Stein, D.J., Benjet, C., Gureje, O., Lund, C., Scott, K.M., Poznyak, V., and van Ommeren, M. (2019). Integrating mental health with other non-communicable diseases. *British Medical Journal*, 364(2019), p. 1295 https://doi.org/10.1136/bmj.l295

Trifu, S., Vladuti, A., and Popescu, A. (2019). The neuroendocrinological aspects of pregnancy and postpartum depression. *Acta Endocrinologica (Bucharest, Romania)*, 15(3), p. 410–415. https://doi.org/10.4183/aeb.2019.410

Weinstein, A.D. (2016). *Prenatal Development and Parents' Lived Experiences – How Early Events Shape Our Psychophysiology and Relationships.* New York: W.W. Norton & Company.

WHO. (2021). What do we mean by self-care? Retrieved from https://www.who.int/ reproductivehealth/self-care-interventions/definitions/en/ [accessed 28.12.21].

Winnicott, D.W. (1953). Transitional objects and transitional phenomena – A study of the first not-me possession 1. *International Journal of Psycho-Analysis*, 24, p. 89–97. Retrieved from https://icpla.edu/wp-content/uploads/2013/02/Winnicott-D.-Transitional-Objects-and-Transitional-Phenomena.pdf [accessed 31.12.2021].

Index

Note: Page numbers in *italics* are figure.